## PRAISE FOR *SUPERPOWERS*

"Noelle Hipke has written a caring, inspirational, and personal book that shares many ideas for readers to consider for improving their well-being. You can hear her voice throughout her journey as she covers everything from nutrition to emotional intelligence. I especially liked her chapter on strategies that touches on so many practical skills we should all study and learn. *Superpowers: A Journey to Self-Health* will make a positive impact on you!"

—Dean Karrel, Career Development Advisor, LinkedIn Learning Instructor, Author of *Mastering the Basics: Simple Lessons for Achieving Success in Business*

"In this fascinating work filled with sage advice, practical tips, and poignant jumping-off points for discussion, Hipke encourages us to develop our extrasensory approach to life and connect with invisible signals and details from the universe. In understanding these hidden elements that we often overlook, we can awaken our superpowers to lead a more harmonious, empowered, and successful life and better know our place within the universe's grand plans.

"Noelle Hipke has crafted a fascinating work from which spiritual readers are sure to take much inspiration. Fans of the nontraditional will enjoy exploring Hipke's well-organized concepts, which are penned using clear, accessible language. I found the journaling opportunities built into the book particularly helpful. This allows us guided reflection and a chance to reshape the advice into ways that best suit our needs.

For example, the section on the digital matrix was interesting to read and a concerning topic in modern times. Hipke's advice on managing digital media and our overreliance on phones is especially practical. It was interesting to hear Hipke's own experiences alongside the direction. The sections where Hipke reflects before and after the activation of her superpowers strike a poignant contrast in a confident narrative tone. *Superpowers* is recommended for anyone seeking nontraditional methods of self-activation and inspiration for change."

—Five-Star Review by K. C. Finn for Readers' Favorite

"*When you are in the middle of a storm, write and release.* Facts, confidences, thoughts, hints, hopes, and dreams[, all] combined in a very appealing literary mosaic[,] present readers with the opportunity to reflect about what really matters in contemporary lives—resilience, self-healing, and self-respect being the actual superpowers which can enable oneself to lead a meaningful existence. Penned by Noelle Hipke's empathetic, loving yet lucid voice, this comprehensive guide to self-discovery can offer readers several aha moments. Hipke's extensive research, added to her storytelling skills, makes great use of literature as an inspirational tool to self-improvement."

—Heloisa Prieto, Best-Selling Brazilian Author of *The Musician*

"The purpose of this book is to provide insight into ways of practicing self-help with an emphasis on self-love. The advice has a positive focus and advocates choosing to listen to your wants and desires instead of what is being told to you by others. At the heart of the book is the concept of finding our superpowers, which are gifts that vary from person to person. This book can be useful for everyone, whether as a spiritual resource, the first steps to self-help, or simply a reminder.

This is a great guide for yoga and meditation enthusiasts as it highlights elements such as the use of the pineal and pituitary glands as superpower activators, learning about the chakras, and the need for clean water.

"The book also doesn't shy away from what is unhealthy for us, such as touching on how to stay hydrated when our water tends to contain chemicals and hormones. This is merely one example of how Noelle Hipke suggests ways to live a healthier life, both mentally and physically. The guide is straightforward with the starting point being how to be aware of different aspects of our lives, such as looking at ways to detox and learning how to identify toxicity. While the book highlights negativity, it focuses on finding the positive, such as identifying important EI qualities (social awareness, self-awareness, senses, and empathy), discovering the different types of learning styles, and how understanding these can be beneficial. This author does not ignore serious topics such as assault, suicide, and drug usage, though it deals with them without judgment and helps people through these situations. *Superpowers* is an extensive resource for those seeking self-care or searching for ways to make a positive change in their lives."

—Five-Star Review by Liz Konkel for Readers' Favorite

"Noelle Hipke's *Superpowers* book could have been titled *Wisdom for the World* because her book is a veritable treasure trove of deep wisdom, wisdom that is needed in our world more than ever before. The post-Covid world is still recovering from the fear propagated by the media, fear that has negatively impacted the health of countless millions of people. Yet in Noelle's marvelous narrative we find a powerful antidote: our superpowers. Latent within us, our superpowers are more powerful that we might imagine, and Noelle guides us in her grounded, refreshingly direct style to release fear, move into love, and rediscover our innate, God-given brilliance, along with the tools and insights needed to attain the vibrant health that is our birthright.

"It is rare that I have read a book in which I found inspiration on almost every page!"

—John Stuart Reid, Acoustic-Physics Scientist, cymascope.com and soundmadevisible.com

"*Superpowers* is a resource for simple steps that are accessible to everyone on a healing journey. Noelle shares what she has discovered with raw honesty into her self-health journey."

—Annette Villaverde, Intuitive Guide, Life Coach, Author

"I have had the honor and privilege of working one on one with Noelle directly. She is the real deal, living what she has written about in this book. In a world that is undergoing a profound shift, Noelle Hipke's *Superpowers* comes as a timely guide for those seeking to awaken their true potential and fulfill their soul's purpose. With remarkable insight and a wealth of knowledge, Hipke takes readers on an illuminating journey of self-discovery and soul healing, unveiling the invisible details of our existence and empowering us to tap into our hidden abilities.

"*Superpowers* not only explores the transformation from a materialistic world to an energetic new earth but also equips readers with the tools to harness their personal frequencies and connect with their higher selves. Through cutting-edge nontraditional methods and concepts, Hipke sheds light on previously ignored aspects of human evolution, inviting us to embrace our unique blueprints and activate our dormant potential.

"What sets *Superpowers* apart is Hipke's ability to weave together profound insights with the stories of luminary visionaries who are working collectively to awaken and heal humanity. The book serves as a rallying cry for individuals to join this conscious collective and contribute to the greater awakening of our world.

"I wholeheartedly recommend *Superpowers* to anyone who seeks to break free from the limitations of the ordinary and step into their extraordinary potential. Noelle Hipke's wisdom, combined with her ability to guide readers through transformative processes, makes this book a powerful tool for those ready to activate their superpowers and ascend to new dimensions."

—Bill McKenna, Founder of Cognomovement, Author of *The Only Lesson*

*Superpowers: A Journey to Self-Health*
by Noelle Hipke

© Copyright 2023 Noelle Hipke

ISBN 978-1-64663-994-6

All rights reserved. No part of this publication may be reproduced, stored in a retrieval system, or transmitted in any form or by any means—electronic, mechanical, photocopy, recording, or any other—except for brief quotations in printed reviews, without the prior written permission of the author.

Published by

◢ köehlerbooks™

3705 Shore Drive
Virginia Beach, VA 23455
800-435-4811
www.koehlerbooks.com

# SUPER POWERS

## A Journey to Self Health

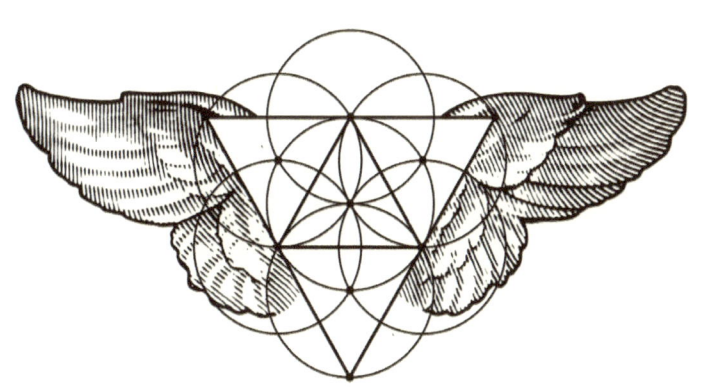

### NOELLE HIPKE

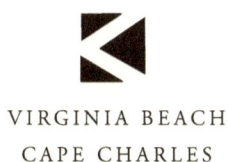

VIRGINIA BEACH
CAPE CHARLES

I dedicate this book to my amazing kids, Westin and Kyra. Without you coming into the world, I would have never had the opportunity to discover who I really am, what I came here to do, and how to become a better role model for you.

To my dad, thank you for being a guardian angel on the other side all these years.

To my guardian angels, it's with deep gratitude that I honor the divine wisdom, knowledge, and enlightenment you have shared with me in my lifetime to assist humanity. Gratitude attitude for your protection and guidance.

To myself, for doing the work and becoming the best version of myself I could ever imagine.

To all souls, beings, and planets in the universe. May you all be happy and free and live lovingly.

## TABLE OF CONTENTS

Introduction ................................................................. 1

**Chapter 1:** The Miracle of Water ................................. 9

**Chapter 2:** Nutrition .................................................. 29

**Chapter 3:** Identity .................................................... 47

**Chapter 4:** The Energetic Body ................................. 93

**Chapter 5:** The Digital Matrix Is Toxic .................... 121

**Chapter 6:** Emotional Intelligence ........................... 138

**Chapter 7:** Strategies ............................................... 154

**Chapter 8:** DNA ...................................................... 201

**Chapter 9:** Healing the Body ................................... 220

**Chapter 10:** Soul Healing ........................................ 282

**Chapter 11:** Wrap-Up .............................................. 306

**Epilogue** ................................................................. 326

**Acknowledgments** ................................................. 328

**References** .............................................................. 329

# INTRODUCTION

After fifty years on this planet, I have realized my "soul" purpose is to help people understand their life's purpose, heal their souls, and tap into their superpowers. Superpowers are extraordinary traits each one of us has. We are all different, and we can see it in our DNA if we know how to analyze it. I am going to teach you how to tap into superpowers that are unique to you.

I have been on a healing journey my entire life, and I have done the work many times over to reinvent myself, heal, realign, and create. I have seen the world change, changed with the world, and observed the past and present, and I always look into the future. I have been planning for my future my entire life. I have set up systems, created concepts, and put into action many items that have served myself, my clients, and my friends and family well. I was met with resistance at times because what I was doing has not been done before, but when the results came, no one could argue. I am a trailblazer. A trailblazer is an innovator who goes off the beaten track to create a new trail. It's not always easy being a trailblazer, because you are ahead of the times and some people are set in their ways. I have been gifted with the superpower of being able to help people feel, comprehend, and put into action steps to align with their higher selves.

I am going to guide you in figuring out what you are good at and what you are here to do. I've spent many years researching, reading, analyzing, and compiling data to understand myself, my children, my family, my friends, and any person I'm considering as a mate. Often, parents project their wants and needs onto their kids by labeling them jock, artist, smart, etc. Parents should not do this until and unless the children have decided for themselves what they will become.

Let's ask questions, research, listen, and look for what makes you light up. This book will teach you how to tap into your superpowers. All I ask is that you keep an open mind. The more open you are to the information, the better you can expand your perspectives and viewpoints as well as opportunities to grow.

As early as twenty years old, I was exploring early insights on life to give me a leg up in my search for who I was; I wanted to interview women of knowledge who were twenty to thirty years older than me, seeking their tips on lessons they'd learned so I could share with others of my generation and use that information to our advantage. I've tried to write this book many times, but I've discovered that when you share your visions with people who can't see it, feel it, or touch it, they will block you from achieving your dreams.

I would tell my mother that I wanted to write a book, and she would respond with, "Now, why would you want to do that? It won't pay the bills." I have binders filled with newsletters, articles, blogs, outlines, poems, and creative writings that poured out of me over the years, but she never saw me as a writer. She has stopped me in my tracks several times due to her beliefs; she does not see, honor, or support my superpower.

It literally took me decades to decide not to listen to her or tell her about this book until it was completed. I am sharing this with you because I want you to understand that other people's fears will hold us back if we let them. And I don't want that to happen to you. Do not let your parents or other people hold you back.

If you to listen to your higher self, you will accomplish everything you have come on this planet to do. Writing this book has been my soul purpose all my life, and I knew it in my early twenties. The big aha moment for me was when I finally ignored everyone else's hang-ups, issues, and fears and chose faith in myself even when they didn't. It felt like getting zapped by lightning when I realized I should be speaking not from other women's viewpoints but from my own personal experiences. I have tracked my experiences, wisdom, knowledge, and research in journals and binders all over my house. I didn't tell anybody anything except that I was fulfilling my "soul purpose." You would be amazed at how excited people got when I told them nothing more than that. I gave very few details, but they could see and feel my energy. People would tell me, "I can't wait to see what you create. This is so exciting!"

My body often tingled as I worked on this book. My cells were singing. That is when I really knew I was following my soul purpose. My soul soared, and the wisdom poured in through universal energy flow. I dreamed of children singing the title of this book and giving me messages about what I was meant to do and the waves of change this book could create for humankind. I soon realized this soul purpose was bigger and brighter than I could have ever imagined. This knowledge has been granted to me as a gift to you. Every lesson, every struggle, every decision, every problem. I could see you all, feel you all, and become one with you all.

I often thought I should have been a therapist, due to my passion for understanding human behavior. It's kind of an addiction. I have worked with healers, coaches, counselors, mentors, and therapists, and have had many of my own healing experiences. And let me tell you, we all are going to need these helpers—all of our lives. Having a therapist is never a bad thing. Mentors can help you get through some of the toughest times in your life. The best way to approach transition is with like-minded people in your court who support, guide, understand, validate, and propel you to the next level.

We are all going to encounter big changes. I have healed myself numerous times from betrayal, divorce, trauma, family issues, toxic people, toxic environments, abuse, alcoholism, and the list goes on. I truly believe I am being guided by the universe to show you how to heal and tap into your superpowers. I type eighty-five words per minute, and the wisdom and information often came faster than I could type. Some days I would turn off my computer and think, *Wow. I can't believe that just came out of me.* I write from my heart to your heart. That is the only way I know how to communicate. So, when you feel my words affecting you, know they were intended just for you.

I made a point of looking at other cultures. I didn't do this much when I was younger, but I learned a lot and expanded my horizons as I got older. By looking at other people's nationalities, cultures, systems, traditions, superstitions, values, and ethics, I found valuable information the average eye can't see if it's not looking for it. When we are young, we don't have a lot of experience to fall back on. This is why the elders in cultures are honored and respected. They have wisdom and link us to our ancestors. We need to learn from our elders in order to keep our lineage alive.

Many people don't treat those of different cultures, beliefs, values, and ethics with respect. We need to change that right now. We must honor and learn from one another. We each value things for different reasons, and those reasons are important to understand. I have noticed that many Americans who do not understand other cultures can be judgmental of them. We are each brought here to earth with our own superpowers, and no two people are alike. Learning about your superpowers and the superpowers of others and discovering your soul purpose will elevate you to accept yourself and others unconditionally.

Think of it as leveling up in a video game. Throughout your life, you will level up as you master karma, life lessons, trauma, and experiences. When you learn the lesson and redirect your attention, you will break the ties that hold you back.

I may repeat myself in this book several times over. I am being directed to say things multiple times because often when you read something only once, the message doesn't stick. I am supposed to give you hints and reminders of what is really important, and you will pick up the rest on your own. I recommend going to the dollar store and getting three to five blank journals. This way you can complete the journal exercises in this book to keep for future reference. You will find the exercises expose patterns, enhance awareness, and alter states of mind to help propel you from one level to the next.

## MY BACKGROUND

In a nutshell, I have been doing yoga since I was fourteen years old and have been connecting to my higher self—also known as intuition—since I was a kid. We all have intuition but often don't understand how to tap into it until we are older. This book is filled with information I wish I'd known when I was younger, and I am passing this knowledge on so you can reap the benefits.

I have been running my own business as a Realtor since 2005 and am a Seniors Real Estate Specialist (SRES), which means I specialize with seniors downsizing and going into senior communities. There's no established method to teach about aging, the process, and what to expect. Seniors go through huge transformations on their way off this planet, and I've learned a lot from witnessing the experience.

I have also gone through large transformations. I went back to college for broadcast journalism in 2014 with kids half my age. I have been taking photos and doing social media and press for the Newport Beach Film Festival since 2010. I knew the future would be worldwide storytelling via the internet, and I wanted to tell my clients' stories like a mini movie. I have been on YouTube since 2008, created my own videos, a web series, websites, and email campaigns, in addition to composing business proposals as well as personalized real estate newsletters for about two decades. I guess you could say I have some experience in the marketing field.

I believe holistic health is the future for humanity. I have worked with some of the best healers in the universe, and many others will surface over the next few years. In 2017 I was led to become a breathwork guide to assist in this transformation. You can create endless possibilities when you align your health and live intentionally. This is the new earth we will be living in. And let me tell you, this near future is going to be one of the best times in history because we are all going to be vibrating at higher levels of consciousness. Controlling and maintaining your energy, vibration and frequency will be of utmost importance as we transition from a materialistic world to an energetic new earth.

I will be hosting webinars and seminars as well as doing personal speaking engagements in order to interact with you all. I plan to bring in some of the best healers I know in the industry to help guide you as well. This is about showing you what you need in order to be *the* highest vibrational version of yourself. Sign up at my website https://NoelleHipke.com to get connected to us and follow us online.

## KINDNESS KICKOFF

I want to share energy with you and truly help you to understand your soul's purpose. We do this by connecting and accepting each other for who we are as individuals.

Use kindness on all levels. Kindness is an invisible superpower if you are not paying attention. Kindness is pure, unconditional love, forgiveness, and acceptance—which is what will change humanity. Have kindness for yourself and others. This in turn will change past, present, and future generations, which means you will ultimately heal your DNA and lineage as you complete this journey.

The goal is to create a healthy, high-vibrational new earth together.
Let our adventure begin.
Be luminary.

*Noelle Hipke*

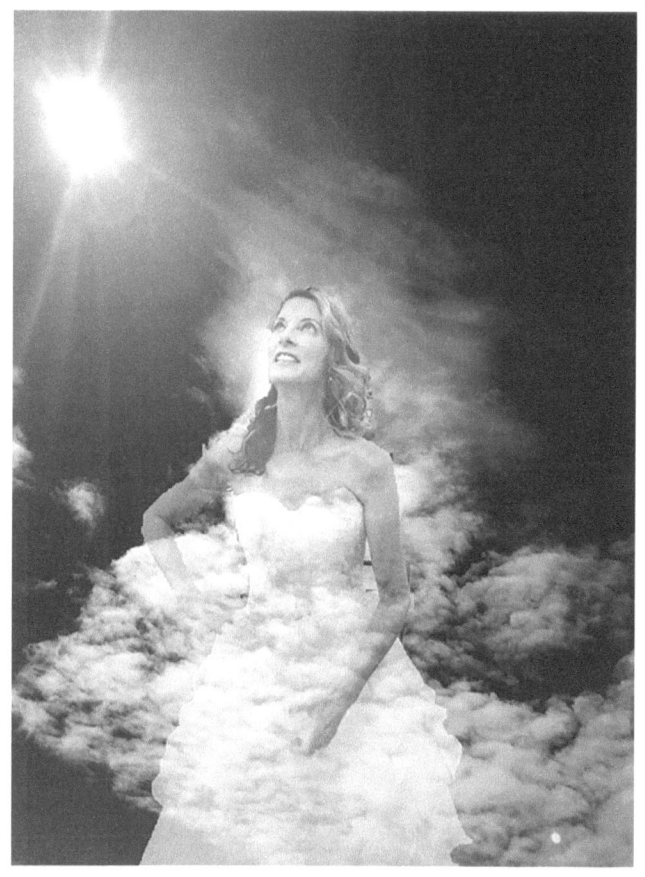

## CHAPTER ONE

# THE MIRACLE OF WATER

Water is life. And it is one of our most precious resources, so don't waste it. Honor it, respect it, and appreciate it. Ever notice how plants, trees, and flowers are brighter, greener, and healthier when watered? Well, that is exactly what happens to our bodies when given the best water on the planet. Maintaining the proper pH levels gives us optimum health. And when we are at our optimum health, we score better on tests and perform better in sports and just about anything we do.

Did you know the body is made up of about 70 percent of water? Water has cosmic energy. It contains cellular life force for our bodies. That means it helps our cells detoxify, clean, hydrate, and thrive and multiply. If your cells don't thrive and multiply, they die off, and you would look like an old person and your organs would stop working properly.

There are certain ways to get the pH level in your body to the right level. Water is by far the best and easiest way to get the result. However, it has to be the right kind of water. Did you know the water in your home contains many contaminants? Pesticides, metals, toxins, and fluoride block the pineal gland. You are drinking and showering with this water. These toxins are all going right into your body, your bloodstream, and your brain.

## PINEAL GLAND

The pineal gland is one of your superpower activators. It is described as the "seat of the soul" and is located in the center of the brain. The main function of the pineal gland is to gather data about the environment and relay this data to produce the hormone melatonin. Melatonin monitors our sleep–wake cycle; it helps regulate your body from sleep to activity. Your pineal gland is also known as your "third eye"—what I call your "invisible information station."

When you change the water you are drinking to pH-balanced, living water, you produce healthy cellular reactions that enable parts of your body to work at an enhanced capability. When you clear the body of toxins and flush out the negative energy, you free up your body in ways you never knew existed.

## PITUITARY GLAND

The pituitary gland is known as the hormone "master gland," stimulating different body functions. This gland picks up what the body needs through the senses and sends signals to the nervous system, toward different glands and organs in the body, monitoring their performance and balancing pH to maintain the body's internal environment.

The water we consume affects how our superpowers are ignited in the body.

Our future is not one of drinking coffee and energy drinks. Our future is drinking the best water we can create on this planet. Why? Because all those chemicals and toxins in alcohol, soda, energy drinks, and coffee limit your superpowers and shut them off. When they are shut off, you are not performing at your best. These beverages give you a surge, but when the surge dies off, you are back to square one, looking for another quick fix. Later in this book, I'll show you how to get a natural quick fix when you need it.

## DR. EMOTO

Okay, here is a fun thing I want you to do. I want you to pull out your electronic device and go to YouTube and look up Dr. Masaru Emoto. This is one of my favorite videos: https://www.youtube.com/

watch?v=FTORSP3uNMA ("Dr. Masaru Emoto - Message from the Water").

The late Dr. Emoto is a Japanese researcher with a PhD in alternative medicine. He has studied, claimed, and proven that human consciousness affects the molecular structure of water, which means our thoughts, intentions, and surroundings could affect the way the water performs in our bodies. Directing energy into water creates results, good or bad. Water responds to words, music, and thoughts. How cool is that?

You can literally activate your superpowers by putting good vibes into the water before you drink it. In one of Emoto's experiments, positive intentions were directed toward water, and it was frozen, creating beautiful snowflakes. Conversely, when negative intentions were directed at water before it was frozen, the crystals looked like shattered glass.

This is what is going through your bloodstream: chaos. Now imagine positive energy going into the body when you drink water. How do you think it would make you feel? Living water is life force.

There are videos on YouTube that teach you how to charge your water. I recommend you check them out to gain a better understanding and discover a personal system that works for you.

## WATER SYSTEMS

I will be sharing with you my very best resources and tips on holistic healing methods. These tried-and-true methods have worked for me as well as many other humans who are leveling up and finding their superpowers.

I have always wanted to put a water filtration system in my house. They are expensive, so I did a lot of research. I called all kinds of installers, seeking a system that would give me the best water on this planet. Many wanted to sell me reverse osmosis, which basically takes everything out of the water, making it pure but not hydrating you. You are drinking clean water, but the water isn't giving anything back to your body.

One of the first things people do when diagnosed with an illness is change their water. I called my healer friend Larisa Stow, who is all about the healing effects of water. She was the one who first told me about Dr. Emoto and the benefits of living water, so I knew she would be a guiding light. You can't put a price tag on your health. Keeping your body clean and clear is going to elevate you to a whole new level.

Larisa told me about a water filtration system she bought called Spring Aqua. I then called the company, and I was connected directly to the owner, Kenny. Kenny and I talked for about an hour. I learned Kenny's family had always been ahead of their time. His godfather developed the Rubik's cube toy as well as his own FDA-approved EKG machine.

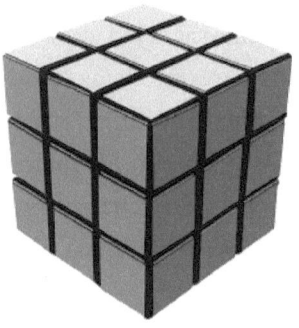
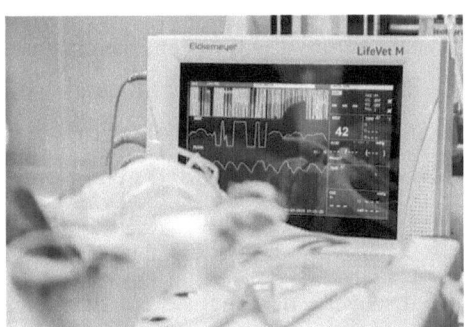

In case you didn't know, the EKG machine is widely used to check people's hearts. Now they even make portable devices that connect to your phone with an app so you can check your own heart.

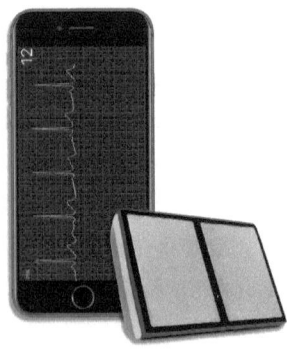

A small tangent: heart attacks are known as a silent killer of women because women are often diagnosed with heart problems later than men and the situation has progressed further. However, women outlive men because they tend to take care of themselves and go in for regular checkups.

Getting back to Spring Aqua: Kenny and his family are operating on a higher vibration and are creating the future in the present. Spring Aqua is not just any water filtration system. Living water offers healing on a cellular level, giving you oxygen, 7.5 and 9.5 pH levels, and supplements to offer healing to the organs and body. This water brings out your superpowers.

Check out all the toxins we currently have in our tap water:

- Chemicals
- Hormones
- Fluoride
- Heavy metals
- Bacteria
- Pesticides

All these toxins block our capabilities to reach our potential. We really need to put a spotlight on this area of our lives. Do not dismiss it! Water connects us to all life forces—food, nutrition, plants, animals, our bodies, and each other.

The water filtration system has eleven to nineteen filters (depending on the system and water where you live) to remove impurities and put in good minerals and supplements in order to mimic natural spring water. The mineral content will vary with the different water sources. This system will first clean the water and allow the good minerals to be ionized and pass through. Then the system will remineralize. One of the minerals they use is called the maifanite stone. Maifan has been used for centuries in Chinese medicine.

Remember: looking at other cultures and integrating their customs allows us to combine resources and create the ultimate soul-healing methods.

Here is a diagram explaining the water elements, the oxygen component, the pH levels, cellular healing and the new, fourth phase of structured plasma for faster absorption. I am honored to bring you the best water filtration system I could find and share the resources.

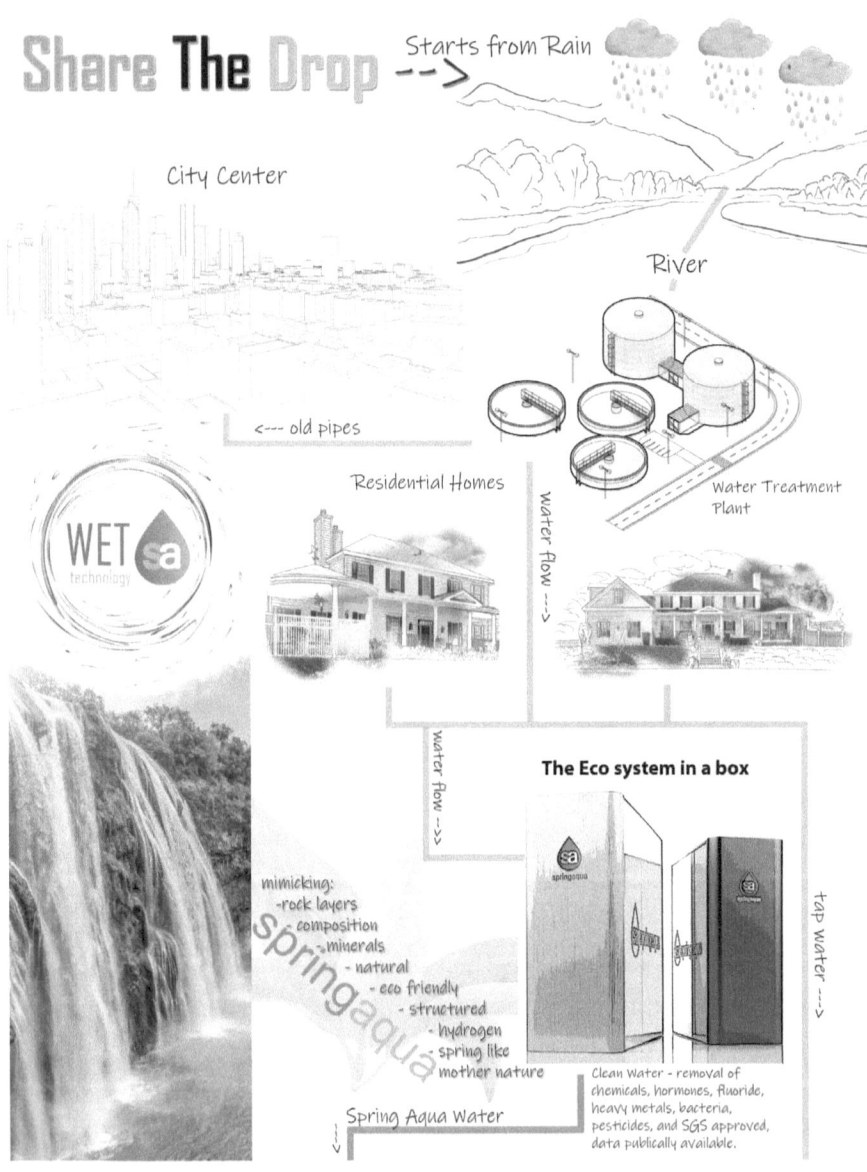

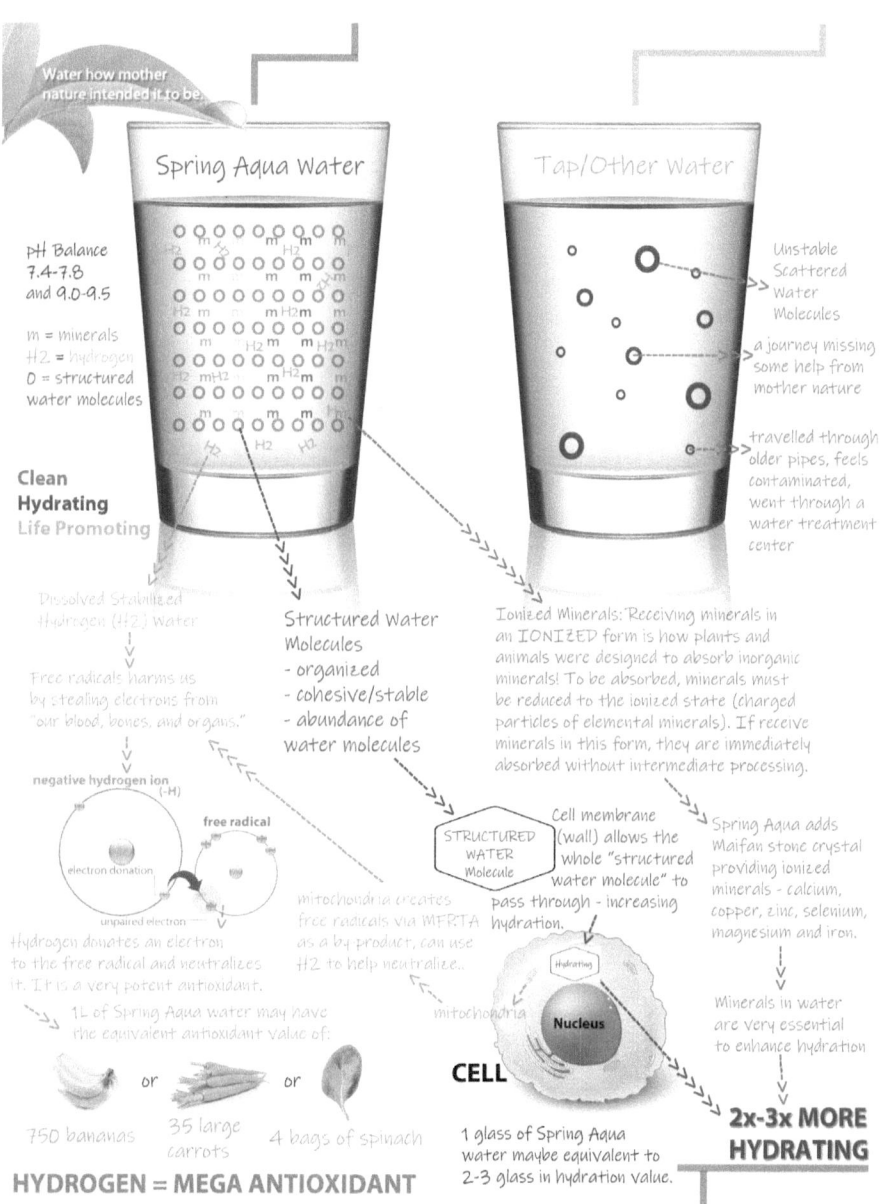

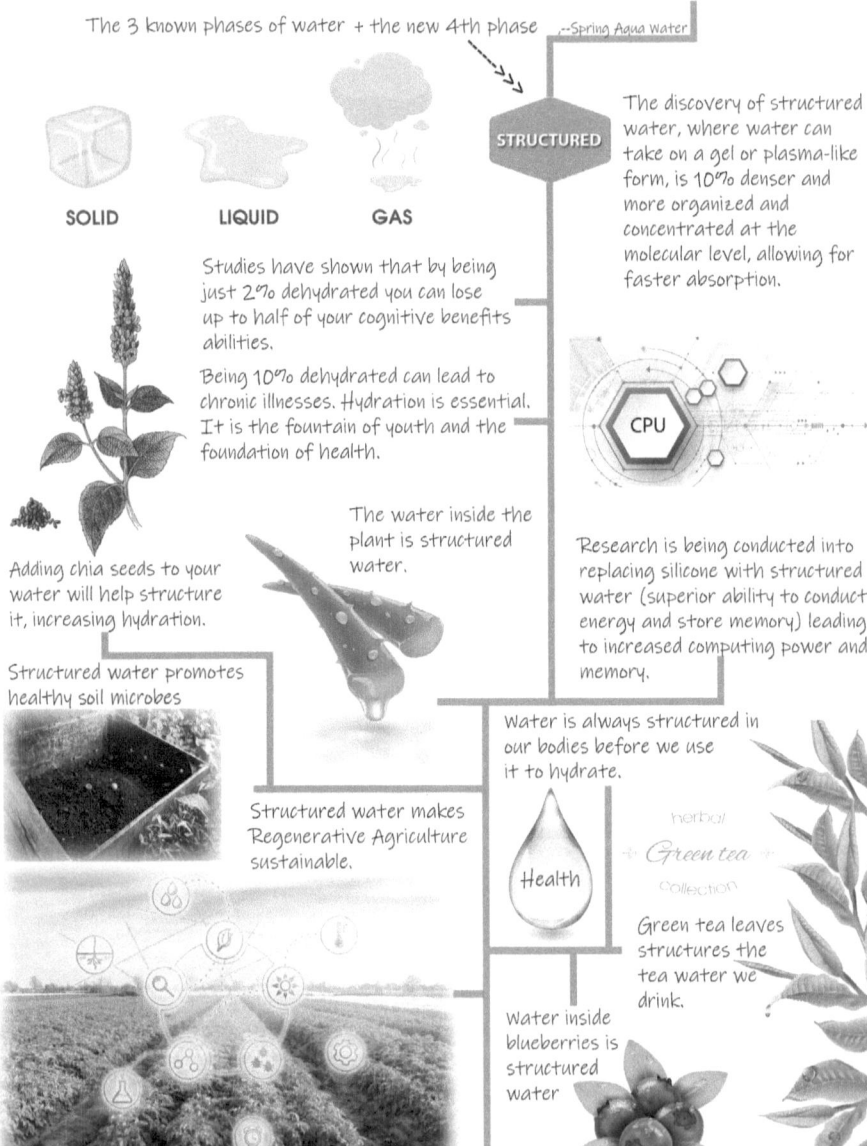

## WATER - WHAT TO KNOW

### What is water?

H2O is only a chemical expression, it does not include any electrical or wave functions. We have now identified a new phase of water: structured. It is a phase beyond vapor, liquid or ice. It is a phase similar to plasma but more organized, in fact so organized that it can actually light up a light bulb. This phase of water can be created in an infrared manner. It is yet another function that is not easily seen in liquid water. The water molecules, in this 4th phase, become so tightly knit that it excludes all contaminants and all other particles of any kind. It is found everywhere and is in fact the phase of water found in every living cell. This discovery has global implications for applications everywhere from health to ecological recovery and computer technology.

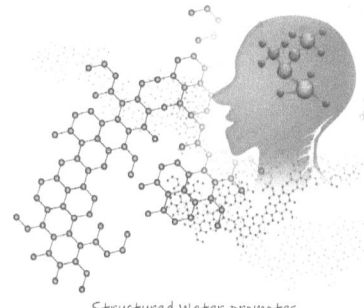

Structured water promotes cell to cell signaling

### What does water do?

Water moistens, but it is so much more than wetness and it runs all biological functions. Hydration and dehydration account for the folding and unfolding of proteins. If there isn't the right kind of water inside of us, all of our functions diminish (muscle, brain, neurological coordination etc). Water is actually life's fuel. It is fuel because water conducts electricity, and we are far more electrical than chemical. Chemicals need electrical ignition to create life. Water is the universal solvent, it disassembles or dissolves all our nutrient molecules, which are not bioavailable until water dissolves them. Water cleanses and carries out waste and contaminants. Without great hydration, we keep all that sludge inside of us. Finally, it is responsible for all cell-to-cell signaling. This is BIG. Water carries and delivers the electrical impulses that dash, dot, dash like morse code. In this way, water is like digital information.

### Water carries information?

Is that what is meant by water has memory? Let me pull the concept of water memory out of all the craziness and set it in clear terms to help us examine this idea. Water memory is the idea that water can carry and pass on molecular information. But water doesn't just pass on information, it stores information so much so that computer scientists are now trying to make quantum computers from water molecules, because water molecules can store more information than silicon. The crystal structure is completely accepted as a storage mechanism and liquid crystals run all of our digital computing. The 4th phase of water, structured water, EZ water, are the many names we have for it now.

**Recommended by Hydration Foundation**

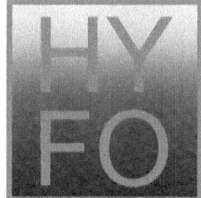

### Dr. Gerald Pollack, who identified this 4th phase water, he say's we are 99% water by molecular count. Is that true?

Scientists are pretty dependent on accurate numbers. Why that number makes sense is that next to hydrogen, the water molecule is the smallest of them all, so it takes a huge volume of those little water molecules to make up all our muscles, our brain, our organs, our eyes, all our tissues. In fact one of the most startling new discoveries is that our connective tissue, called fascia, is actually made up of water in gel like form, stretched out like cobwebs. Like sonogram or EKG gel, this form of jelly or plasma like concentration conducts electricity at a far better rate than liquid water. That makes our connective tissue an information network in our body. We are made up of so much water and information we are only now understanding how profound that is.

*Clean, Hydrating and Life Promoting.*
The way mother nature intended it to be.

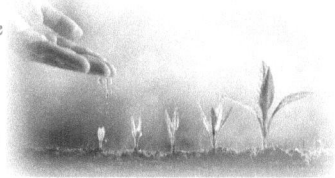

Here is the really cool thing I want to share with you. The maifanite stone adds the following back into the system:

- Magnesium
- Calcium
- Zinc
- Selenium
- Copper
- Iron
- Trace elements

All the trace elements combined total about twenty-six micronutrients. Spring Aqua is structured, clean (certified by SGS), and has cellular life, combining benefits of minerals, hydrogen, regular water, and alkaline water. Spring Aqua is supported and recommended by Organic Healthy Life and the Hydration Foundation. How is that for amazing awareness support?

Spring Aqua creates natural spring water you would find in nature. I love this. Let's cover what some of the minerals do for our bodies:

- Magnesium: supports muscle and nerve function and energy production. Magnesium has many benefits: it creates reactions in your body from biochemicals; boosts exercise performance; combats depression; supports healthy blood sugar levels and a healthy heart; boosts anti-inflammatory benefits, helping prevent headaches (many headaches are caused by lack of water); and regulates PMS symptoms. Constant low levels of magnesium can increase the risk of type 2 diabetes, high blood pressure, heart disease, and osteoporosis.
- Calcium: maintains and builds strong bones. Your nerves, muscles, and heart need calcium to function and operate properly. Benefits: lowers risk of high blood pressure and improves cholesterol values. Some studies suggest that vitamin

D in addition to calcium benefits our bone health and may protect against high blood pressure, cancer, and diabetes.

- Zinc: helps your metabolism and immune system function. Zinc is present in every cell in your body and is needed for the activity of over 300 enzymes that assist in digestion, nerves, metabolism, and several other body functions. Our bodies depend on it for cell growth and division. Zinc is important for healing wounds and assists in your senses of smell and taste. It also alleviates oxidative stress by boosting the activity of T-cells and natural killer cells, which help protect your body from infections. Benefits: immunity, gene expression, enzymatic responses, synthesizing of proteins, DNA synthesis, developing, and growing. People with acne, a common skin disease estimated to affect up to 9.4 percent of the global population, tend to have lower levels of zinc.

  Causes of zinc deficiency include malnutrition caused by anorexia or bulimia, Crohn's disease, gastrointestinal disease, vegetarianism, pregnancy and breastfeeding, sickle cell anemia, kidney disease, or alcohol abuse.

- Selenium: helps to make DNA and protect against cell damage and infections. Selenium is necessary for proper thyroid hormone production. These hormones work with our metabolism, which transforms the food you put into your body into energy. This energy is processed internally to keep many of the body's systems working properly. Close to ten million Americans age eighteen or older are likely to have a thyroid medical issue. It is especially dominant among women: around 10 percent of women may have a thyroid hormone deficiency. Millions in the US are suffering from hypothyroidism right now and don't know even know it.

  System depressants like alcohol, smoking, and stress can cause an overabundance of free radicals in the body. Oxidative stress impairs and damages healthy cells and has therefore been linked to premature aging, chronic conditions like cancer, heart disease, and Alzheimer's, and the risk of stroke. Selenium can reduce the risk of certain diseases, ward off mental decline, boost immunity, reduce asthma symptoms, and intercept DNA damage.

- Copper: assists in the development of energy, tissues, and blood vessels. It balances the immune and nervous systems while activating our genes and aids in brain development. Benefits: creates red blood cells, maintains healthy nerve cells, supports the immune system and formation of collagen—an important protein for your skin, tissues, and bones and defending them from cell damage. Copper helps your body absorb iron, transforms sugar into energy, defends against osteoporosis and arthritis, promotes a healthy heart, and is an antioxidant. Copper imbalance has been linked to Alzheimer's disease, which is one of the number one killers in America.

- Iron: needed for developing and growing. Iron helps construct hemoglobin, an important protein contained in red blood cells. This protein supports oxygen to the muscles and every single part of the body. Iron promotes focus, energy, gastrointestinal operation, the immune system, and body temperature regulation. Iron is necessary for the production of hormones. Symptoms of iron deficiency include pale skin, chest pain, headaches, fatigue, weakness, fast heartbeat, dizziness, chilled hands and feet, brittle nails, and weird cravings for non-nutritive substances, such as dirt, starch, or ice.

Let me point out the importance here of taking a multivitamin no matter what your age. We don't eat right 100 percent of the time, so let's cover our bases. If you think all these health issues won't happen to you because you are still young, think again. The world and environment is working against our bodies; we should take the extra measures to combat them.

Modifying intake of food, adding supplements, and listening to our bodies is part of the puzzle. We know what feels right. How do we know? Ask your body, ask yourself, and listen. Now is the time to spread the word about how vital living water can be. You will vibrate at a higher level. Those living components in the water bring out your superpowers.

I encourage you to do the research and learn more about the water you consume in your community and the water filtration systems out there.

More info on Spring Aqua can be found at https://springaqua.info/wellnesswater or https://www.LuminaryHealingCenter.com. If you contact Spring Aqua directly, please let them know Noelle Hipke shared this information with you. A percentage of the money generated from the purchase of this filtration system will be donated to the fight against human trafficking.

• • •

# DETOXIFICATION

## Getting Clear

In order to really get clear, intentional, and focused, you need to rid the body of all toxins at all costs. Detoxification removes impurities in the body, giving you direct connection to your superpowers. When I cleaned out my body, I radiated, my mind was ultra-clear, and I could sense things like I never had before.

Remove these toxins:

1. Alcohol
2. Marijuana
3. Drugs
4. Sugar and processed foods

Reduce intake of these:

1. Salt
2. Wheat
3. Dairy
4. Meats

I know this doesn't sound fun, but once you create a good habit, the positive program is set. You will find it well worth the effort and investment when you realize how much money you save, the better choices you make, how good you feel, and your ability to use your superpowers. Eventually, you won't miss the bad foods; your superpowers will far outweigh your short-term enjoyment of them, and later in this book I will explain and share with you exactly why. Once you tap into your superpowers, you will never want to go back.

What are the benefits of detoxification?

- Fertility: if you want to have children, this is where you should start.
- Purification of blood
- Reduced internal inflammation, which affects your body, tissues, joints, bones
- Better sleep
- Better clarity and focus, focus, focus
- Boosted circulation, inducing accelerated healing
- Boosted energy
- Weight loss
- Stronger immune system
- Improved skin
- Better breath
- Healthy hair

- Lighter feeling
- Anti-aging benefits
- Improved sense of well-being
- Heightened senses

These benefits are amazing. When you get used to living in alignment, you really notice when you are not. Starting off slow is fine, and when you get your routine, throw it into high gear and create your new lifestyle.

Detoxing is the king of spring cleaning. A study conducted by the Environmental Working Group on newborn babies found over 200 toxins in the babies' blood when they were born. That is not good news. We are subjected to toxins in the body each and every day—in the air we breathe, the food we eat, the drinks we consume, and the products we use on our bodies. They build up through vaccines, medications, electronics, and cleaning products as well. There is no escaping. So, what can we do to combat this daily issue? Put the right products in our bodies, for starters, and take the necessary steps to flush out our system on a regular basis. Having good water with which to flush is a crucial part of activating your superpowers.

Detoxing is done through a combination of flushing, juicing, supplements, and fasting. When you trigger your body to use its resources and flush out the toxins, you experience an enlightened sensation, activating super senses in the body.

Here are the benefits I received when I did a detox system:

- Weight loss
- Muscle mass gain
- Flatter stomach
- Tighter skin
- Glowing skin
- Less wrinkles

- Mental clarity
- Stronger immunity
- Increased strength
- Increased stamina
- Sleeping through the night
- Heightened senses
- Superpowers ignited

## Cleaning Products

With regard to cleaning products, something my parents never told me that I will tell you is to always wear cleaning gloves when using household products to clean your home, your office, your bathroom, etc. And I would also consider wearing a mask. Better yet, buy safe cleaning products and get ahead of the problem. These are things we are not told and don't think about. But those chemicals go right into your bloodstream when you handle them. Nothing is safe; your body is going to respond to it eventually. Why put unnecessary strain on your system when you can avoid it all together?

## Nutritional Reset: Detoxing Metals

Here's something that not everyone realizes: Our bodies have accumulated many metals over years of drinking the wrong water, eating the wrong foods, using toxic products, and breathing polluted air. This buildup in our bodies causes brain fog, Alzheimer's disease, infertility, hormone imbalances, and a glut of other health issues. By flushing the metals out of the body, you remove the issue on a cellular level, so finding a detox program that removes metal toxins from the body is key. So far, I have only come across one product that offers this benefit: fulvic zeolite.

A nutritional reset can help naturally remove toxins as well as metals. Considering that an estimated 25 percent of vaccines and flu shots contain a mercury-based preservative, this is a really big deal. Mercury affects the central nervous system, kidneys, liver, and can disturb the immune process, as well as cause impaired vision and hearing, tremors, paralysis, insomnia, and emotional instability. Mercury is going to blow out your superpowers, so eliminating and removing it will work in your favor. We really have to pay attention to what we are putting into and doing to our bodies.

This section makes for a good transition into the next chapter regarding nutrition. A nutrition-based detoxification reset system has helped people lose weight, lose belly fat, gain muscle, clear the mind, and activate other amazing capabilities. Many elderly people suffer from lack of nutrition and hydration because they lose the sensations that lead them to desire nutrients and water, which in turn makes them weak and fragile through bone loss and lack of collagen. The natural nutritional products I've come across have been in the making for over twenty years, using the finest herbs on the planet.

By utilizing supplements and protein shakes with unusual herbs that enable our body to self-heal, we elevate our bodies on a cellular level. I use protein shakes in conjunction with living water, and the benefits are off the charts.

A nutritional reset offers a wide variety of benefits you won't find anywhere else:

- Antioxidants
- Phytochemicals supporting healthy joints
- Better metabolism
- Healthy skin, hair and nails
- Deeper sleep
- Defense against free radical damage
- Anti-inflammation
- Decrease in visible signs of aging
- Defense against oxidative damage of UVA radiation

- Better energy levels, digestion, and mood
- Gut health supported by vegan protein, greens, healthy fats, organic super fruits
- Nutritional support system
- Allergy reduction
- Better endurance and stamina
- Better thyroid, organ, heart, and brain health
- Hormonal balance
- Nutrition for kids and pets

## Spirulina

Have you ever heard of the herb spirulina? Well, I never had until I found natural nutritional products.

Benefits of spirulina:

1. Extremely high in nutrients: protein, B1, B2, B3 vitamins, copper, iron
2. Powerful antioxidant and anti-inflammatory: oxidative damage can harm your DNA and cells
3. Lowers "bad" cholesterol: heart disease is the world's leading cause of death
4. Anti-cancer properties
5. Reduces blood pressure
6. Improves symptoms of allergies
7. Effective against anemia, a decrease in red blood cells
8. Improves muscle strength and endurance
9. Controls blood sugar

I am impressed by the extensive research and the organic extremes nutritional reset programs have undertaken to create the healthiest method they could possibly produce—right down to the recyclable containers. Nutritional products and supplements assist with many health ailments. I integrated the best products I could find and went off the thyroid medicine I had been using for ten years. My skin changed for the better in terms of texture, color, and elasticity. Products are focused on all health areas, including kids and pets.

My goal is not to sell you products but to help you, hear you, see you, and educate and guide you to the right resources to generate a personal health transformation. I recommend a nutritional reset as a starting point when you enter your healing journey. Please check out my website at https://www.LuminaryHealingCenter.com and set up a consultation so you can be guided and supported properly.

. . .

## WELLNESS REMINDERS

- The future is not about coffee, energy drinks, and alcohol.
- The future is about drinking water with the right pH levels, electrolytes, minerals, and supplements.
- Having a water bottle with affirmations—health, happiness, love, energy, or whatever superpowers you want to promote—is "in."
- Loving your body and loving yourself gives you the best health.
- Detoxification is the answer.

> **JOURNAL: Chapter 1**
>
> 1. What are all the benefits you will receive from drinking living water?
> 2. What are the benefits of detoxifying the body?
> 3. List the minerals in our living water and what it does for our bodies. What do the minerals combat?

If interested in researching or learning more, check out https://www.LuminaryHealingCenter.com. Please let any of the resources you contact directly know that Noelle Hipke referred you. This way we can donate a part of the proceeds to combat human trafficking.

## CHAPTER TWO

# NUTRITION

Nutrition is something my parents never talked to me about. I grew up eating Ding Dongs, popcorn, candy, chips, and soda, just to name a few. When walking home from school, a friend and I would stop by the grocery and grab a bag of Doritos, chocolate chip cookie dough, and a soda to wash it down. It was our daily ritual.

My mom cooked from scratch pretty much every night because we didn't have a lot of money. When the microwave became a hot appliance in the 1970s, it changed the way we cooked. Meals were now made in a few minutes instead of thirty or more.

When I became a parent, I wasn't knowledgeable about nutrition. I had a panic attack when the microwave in our home broke. How was I supposed to cook a meal for a family of four without a microwave? We quickly went to the store and bought a replacement, only to discover I didn't like the way it functioned. So I sent my very ticked-off then-husband to return it and purchase a better name brand, which I still have to this day.

In time, as I became savvy that my body was in need of something else, I did research. I was gravitating toward a more holistic, natural healthy lifestyle and discovered that microwaving is actually one of the unhealthiest ways to cook food. Microwaves do things to the food that takes the nutrients out. That was when I started paying more attention to everything. I read more labels and purchased organic everything: fruits, veggies, milk, and eggs. I removed microwave popcorn, mac and cheese, and pretty much anything else that required microwave cooking from my diet. I used to microwave water for a hot cup of tea—what an idiot.

My body had been screaming at me, "Wake up woman! This isn't working." Ironically, my mother-in-law went to school for nutrition and never said one word to me. She never discussed how to improve and eat better. So I think it is really important to mention that the only person you should trust to think about your nutrition is *you*. Your nutrition is what activates your superpowers. What you put in your body is the body's fuel. Food is medicine. Food is energy.

## WAKE-UP CALL

I had a friend who was fighting breast cancer. She asked me one day to take her to get a blood transfusion. I drove her to the hospital, and we entered a large, square room with big windows letting in natural light. Twenty-five La-Z-Boy-type chairs outlined the perimeter. The room was filled with patients receiving IV fluids in their arms or hands. It was a sight I will never forget. My heart sank when I realized the ramifications.

I was directed to sit in another room while I waited for my friend to receive her transfusion. Thank God. I don't think I could have handled witnessing that situation for long. During my wait, so many things reeled through my head. She was my first friend to have cancer. And the sight I saw made me so scared for her. I started to imagine what must have been going through her head and body.

For years she was treated poorly by her husband, who cheated on her, and her teenage son, who disrespected her—a very hostile, toxic environment. She was an amazing writer for a top soap opera magazine, at times surrounded by famous people. I had met her at a church during Bible study. She was a ray of light, inside and out—peppy, positive, energetic, smart, and fun. When I went to her house one day, I asked her about the type of food she consumed. I mentioned that I had switched to buying organic foods a few years back and asked if she was doing the same.

She said, "No, it costs too much."

And I said, "No. What costs too much is bad health."

It is worth the investment to buy the best organic items you can find. And if you can't buy them, grow them yourself.

In time, I watched her lose her hair, her eyelashes, and her eyebrows and dwindle as she underwent radiation treatments. Her husband left her, and she ended up renting out a room in her home and struggled to make it. Her sister, who was in her early thirties, had been the first one diagnosed with breast cancer after testing negative three times. The sister knew something was not right, went into the doctor insisting on a biopsy and the doctor essentially laughed at her. He thought she was too young to worry and brushed it off.

However, she refused to leave until they did a biopsy (examination of tissue removed). Sure enough, her biopsy showed cancer. Turns out my friend, her sister, and her mom all had breast cancer at one point in their lives. Years later they discovered that family members in another country had suffered the same hardship and now they are doing a medical study on their entire family.

This is why *you* need to pay attention to what your body is trying to communicate. You will be way more attuned than some judgmental doctor. Your higher self will guide you; it's like a voice that whispers. And if you don't feel like you've received the answers you needed, get another opinion. Doctors don't know everything. They are just guessing from the symptoms you report. They can't feel you like you do.

I am happy to say my friend recovered from her illness and met a man with three great kids, and she ended up marrying him and taking the children on as her own. In the end, she was gifted a wonderful family who adores her.

I truly believe her environment, the negative energy, the lack of nutrition, and toxic mindset had a huge effect on the severity of her health situation. She altered her life, turned it around, and won in the end.

## NUTRITION COACH: AYURVEDA ALCHEMY

I believe we all should work with a nutrition specialist when it comes to honing our health. It's almost impossible to figure out everything that is or is not good for our bodies without the help of an expert. What we should eat is determined by what our DNA needs. As kids, we are told to drink milk and eat dairy and grains—only to now discover that many of these foods can't be digested properly and should be consumed in moderation or cut out completely.

I couldn't get my thyroid in alignment. Being a bit of a yogi, I hired an Ayurveda nutritionist. This was one of many times that I went to another culture for their expert guidance rather than listening to just anybody. Ayurveda dates back 5,000 years to India and is the world's oldest health system. Food is considered medicine in Ayurveda.

Ancient Eastern health wisdom in conjunction with modern Western nutrition can create a healthy lifestyle in true alignment with you, your body, and your DNA. Bottom line: Ayurveda detects bio-individuality. Every single being is genetically different from every other being. We should likewise feed and treat each of our bodies in a unique way.

The woman I hired, Sandhiya Ramaswamy, gave me eleven pages to fill out. She was asking for *a lot* of history on me: illnesses, hospitalizations, operations, my appetite, my digestion, elimination, sweat, skin, sleep, body temp, mental issues, focus, attitude, moods, decision-making, speech, emotions, mental feelings, family history, cancer, diabetes, blood pressure, pregnancy (how many were successful vs. unsuccessful), PMS, childhood upbringing, menopause, physical and psychological and emotional health challenges, health goals, current habits, intake of caffeine and tobacco and alcohol and drugs, exercise, and routines.

She wanted to know what organic foods I consumed, how often I ate out, if I liked to cook, eating patterns, allergies, dislikes. She even wanted to know my sex level, stress level, and energy level, and what medications, herbs, and supplements I was on. This woman dissected the heck out of me. Never in my life had a doctor asked all these questions, and I still have the eleven-page history to this day. We then proceeded to do a Zoom call so she could take a look at me. She wanted to see the shape of my body, the structure of my face, eyes, and mouth, and my skin texture; she even asked me to stick out my tongue. What was she gonna do next? Look up my butt?

This is what I learned: In Ayurveda alchemy, you have a blueprint of your true nature. Sandhiya figured out my blueprint by reading between the lines and looking at me from the inside out. What we put in our mouths shows on the outside. Your skin is the biggest organ on your body, so if you want to look young and be healthy, you need to pay attention to this part.

There are three main mind–body types, known as doshas, in Ayurveda—Vata, Pitta, and Kapha. Vata is thin, Pitta is medium, and Kapha is larger built. We each have a bit of each one in us, depending on the seasons, and some are more dominant than the others.

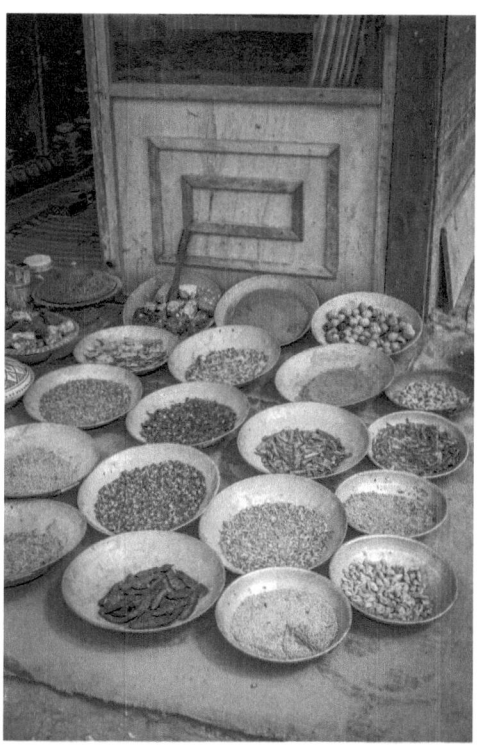

The goal is to fill in the gaps of the ones we are lacking. We do this by adding supplements, oils, spices, herbs, and certain foods. There are also foods we want to avoid. For me, popcorn sucked up all the water in my body, and mushrooms made me sleepy. I needed to stay away from bubbly drinks and consume warm soups, teas, and meals to keep my body digesting foods properly.

I instantly noticed a difference in my skin, feelings, mood, and mindset. The fact that food is considered medicine in Ayurveda makes complete sense since food controls your body, mind, organs, and overall functioning. Consuming healthy, organic food should be your top priority. By aligning with your nutritional essence, you can access your superpowers.

## FREQUENCIES

When you activate your superpowers, you can sense things many other people can't see or understand. Your vibrational frequency will accelerate. That is how a lot of athletes make their magic happen. They align with their higher self, set the intention, eat the right foods to give their body the best fuel, and then intentionally create exactly what they are meant to do. And you can do the same every day. You just have to steer clear of alcohol, drugs, and toxins—basically anything that will jack up your neurological alignment.

So much data is flying around, and you don't even know it. This invisible information goes into your body and third eye, or what I've called the invisible information station. You might not see people's third eye on the forehead above their physical eyes, but it's there. It's gathering data on you, around you, and through you energetically and filing it away. If you think a white lie won't be detected, think again. Our bodies constantly give off signals unconsciously. We humans have the capability to feel things on the other side of the planet—and most likely the universe—if we are paying attention. (When is the last time you looked up at that big sky? You can't possibility believe we are the only beings in the universe, can you?)

Flying high as a kite on your own vibrational frequency while sensing others' vibrational frequencies is what being in your superpowers means. This may explain why a lot of people can't get along. People who don't eat well or don't take care of themselves can make you feel funky. Those vibrational frequencies are so different and unaligned with your own that being around them can feel draining or irritating. They are energy vampires, sucking the life force energy out of you to make up for the energy they are missing.

I found myself moving away from certain friends when I started to vibrate higher. I worked hard to get to a high frequency. I sure as heck wasn't going to let them take me down with them. I cannot control the choices they make, only my own.

## SCHOOL DISTRICTS

One day, my daughter's school district had a pre-screening for the parents to watch the videos that would be shown to our kids in reference to puberty. Being an older, wiser woman, I took my ten-year-old, fifth-grade daughter to the screening. I was about to start on this book and wanted to be sure of what they were teaching the children.

I was the only parent who showed up with their kid in tow. Quite frankly, in the beginning the other parents and administration were concerned about why I had brought her at all. There were only about eight of us in the room, and of course we had to sit in the front row so my daughter could get the best view.

They showed videos that were twelve to fifteen years old. The only thing the video mentioned about nutrition was to drink water and milk and not a lot of soda. And get this: the plan was that the girls would go into one room and view the girls' video, and the boys would go into another room and view the boys' video *only*. Which meant the boys and girls never got to see the videos about the opposite sex and how their bodies changed. Say what? My daughter giggled through the boys' video, and the other parents in the room were upset their kids would not see the opposite-sex video and wondered where they might be able to find it to show to their kids.

I'd done this rodeo before with another kid who is now twenty-three, and I wasn't nearly as aware of and involved with teaching the tools of life as I am today. As a young parent, you don't think about some of these things until much later in life. And if your parents didn't teach them to you, you might never know them at all. My second child benefited a lot from lessons learned; and now so will you. If each school had a nutritionist on hand to guide kids and create a custom nutrition plan, this would give our kids the superpower education they need to fulfill their wishes and dreams on their own terms.

Your nutrition is unique, just like you. I highly recommend hiring your own nutritionist so you can create a custom plan generated just for you and your body. It is the best gift you can give yourself for *life*.

## JUICING

Check out the film *Fat, Sick and Nearly Dead*. After watching that film, I turned to juicing. Juicing eliminated a lot of the toxins in my body, and I had a rather beautiful glow in my aura afterward. My skin looked amazing, my eyes were clear, my feelings were good—heck, I *radiated*. I could see it and feel it, and other people noticed something was different. Juicing is like putting the good stuff right into your bloodstream with an IV. What is not to love about this?

I have now gone through three juicers in my lifetime and recently splurged on the best name brand I know. It is worth the price to invest in yourself and your health. People think all they need is healthcare insurance, when in reality you need the tools and info to take care of your body to the best of your abilities. Consider this a personal instruction booklet on how to care for yourself. I strongly encourage you to work with a health coach. Mine told me to add certain veggies, such as carrots and beets, to the juice mix to give me that extra oomph my body needed.

Juice Recipe: 2 green apples, 1 lemon, 1 cup spinach, 1 cup kale, 1 cucumber, 1 beet, 4 carrots, slice of ginger.

## HOAG HOSPITAL: THE WEALTHY HOSPITAL

One day in 2018, I found myself on a first date in Newport Beach, California, at the Balboa Yacht Club. Newport Beach is one of the richest cities in the Orange County area where I live, so its population is considered high society. Upon meeting my date, he whisked me away onto this majestic yacht. I was the only woman sitting in a circle of men: the head physician of Neurology at Hoag Hospital, anesthesiologists, neurosurgeons, and my date, Mr. Stem Cell Guy. I found out they were in a band together, and my guy was the lead singer.

I soon turned into the new entertainment since I was the new kid on the block and the only female. I held my own by being savvy, informed, confident, and wise. In most cases, I think a woman would be intimated by this situation. But not me. I've always known that if you can network with people of status, power, and connections, you can get anything done. I was offered a cocktail beverage, and I requested water, stating I don't drink. The head of Neurology was curious. I proceeded to state that I am into holistic health and I think it is the wave of the future. To my surprise, the head physician agreed. He said that anytime a new patient came to him, he had them start with changing their nutrition. It turned out his wife was a nutritionist, and she didn't drink either.

So there. I'm already doing what some of the wealthiest people on the planet are paying a small fortune for someone else to tell them to do. But is anybody telling our kids? That is where it needs to start so we can help the next generations. This is yet another reason why I am writing this book.

As for Mr. Stem Cell Guy, he was overweight and used food as a crutch and reward. On our second date, he practically moved right into my house and told me how much his mom was going to love me.

*Thanks for the compliment, but you gotta go now; we are not in lifestyle alignment.* These were low-vibration issues I did not want in my life, so I shooed him away.

## INTEGRATIVE HEALTH

At one point in my life, I saw an integrative health specialist for my thyroid issue. Integrative health coordinates holistic and traditional care. The integrative health specialist cost me about $500 a visit between bloodwork, supplements, and her consultation fee. This type of healthcare isn't usually covered by health insurance.

I wasn't ready to give up drinking alcohol and change my diet back then. I struggled mentally, emotionally, and physically for quite some time, trying to get on track. I spent thousands of dollars trying her methods, which didn't seem to work. When I look back on it, I realize I was in a toxic relationship with myself; I was not willing to do the necessary work to gain my health back, like stop drinking alcohol or change my diet. Those choices prevented me from healing.

You have to be willing and able to make the necessary changes and embrace it as your new lifestyle in order to be successful. There is no temporary fix. Make it a permanent lifestyle change, and you will reap the benefits for life.

## RED MEAT

In 2016, I had been on Accutane for acne twice in my lifetime. I heard my higher self whisper, *Get off red meat. The hormones and antibiotics in them are wreaking havoc on your system.* I made the decision to stop eating red meat, and within six months, my entire life and skin changed dramatically for the better.

There is something I want you to think about here. Animals are pumped with antibiotics to get them to grow fast and prevent illness, and pesticides are used on the foods animals eat, while red meat itself is high in cholesterol, saturated fats, and sodium (salt). All this is going directly into your system when you eat the meat. In addition, these animals are contained to be slaughtered for food consumption, and they know what is happening. They understand the environment through their senses, just like we do. So these animals are basically living in fear.

When you consume the animal, you consume all of these energies.

## MENSTRUAL CYCLES

Children are consuming foods that stimulate fertility at a premature age. Many girls are getting their periods as early as eight. This in turn shortens the window of time in which they can bear children. This is really important to pay attention to as it could affect our ability to populate the planet. A lot of soil has also lost its nutrients over the years, so this could affect our food. If too many factors are tampered with, women of the future could have a very difficult time bearing children.

I didn't start my period until I was seventeen years old. I was the fourth generation in my family to bear children in my forties. I believe this was due to the fact that I started my menstrual cycle at a later age, granting me more eggs over a longer period of time. The food we were eating back then wasn't ultra-healthy relative to what we know now, but in the 1970s and 1980s, we weren't bombarded with the toxins we are today. I have made the extra effort to give my daughter the best organic products to keep her healthy and thriving for the long run. I want to share this with you so you can see the patterns that are appearing.

## BUILD A GARDEN

I truly believe building and maintaining our own private vegetable and fruit gardens is the wave of the present and future. If we can supply for ourselves the items we enjoy and grow them with love, we can create the healthiest vibration for ourselves and our families. Putting love into the food we grow and cook is like putting love directly into our bodies. We radiate and become more love. Who wouldn't want that?

When I was in New Zealand in 2014 and 2016, I noticed many people grew their own fruits and veggies; for meals, they would go out into their yard, pluck food off the vine, and put it right into the dish they were eating that very moment. That food was superpowered. Why? Because it didn't lose any nutrients from being packaged, shipped, and placed on the shelf in the store. By the time we get our food, it has lost a lot of healing qualities. We need to coordinate agriculture classes in our areas to help people learn how to cultivate the land and grow their own fruits and veggies. There are even systems for growing food plants on balconies if that is the only space you have.

I met a man in his sixties who was given six months to live due to an illness. Upon diagnosis, he chose to go completely vegan. He started growing his own fruits and veggies and changed his lifestyle for the better. He has now outlived two of his doctors and is still thriving over a decade later. I introduce this man as Farmer Phil, and he loves sharing his passion and expertise on how to build edible gardens. He is always offering his healing foods of love to friends and neighbors.

Building your own garden is one of the best gifts of love you can give yourself. Putting love into the food and then taking that food into yourself makes you pure, radiant love. Fruits and veggies are here on this planet for a reason. Eat them and activate your superpowers. Glow get it.

## WHAT TO EAT?

In order to leave you well equipped to instantly take charge of your nutrition, I am going to give you some basic ideas about what you can consume as a general guideline until you find a nutrition coach to work with.

- Shop fresh, local, and whole.
- Consume natural grass-fed meats with no antibiotics.
- Consume farmed fresh fish, seeking low-mercury fish.
- Steer clear of grains and all gluten, or consume moderately.

- Look for items with no or low pesticides, no antibiotics, no hormones, no chemicals, no additives, no preservatives.
- Eat organic fresh fruits and vegetables.
- Use a juicer for juicing to get instant results.
- Nuts are a great option for healthy snacks if you are not allergic.
- Try to eliminate or reduce intake of dairy products, processed fats, acidic foods, and animal flesh.

Find a nutritionist as soon as you possibly can. Get tested for allergies if necessary. You need to learn the right type of gas to put into your special car. The quality of the food you eat will affect how you feel about your life.

## TRANSFORM YOUR LIFE WITH SUPPLEMENTS

What I discovered on my journey is that we need supplements to fill in the gaps. Sometimes we can't get enough of the right ingredients from food alone. Some herbs and superfoods can help propel our bodies to the next level.

Many people have gut issues from antibiotics, which work against our bodies and create internal problems. Finding a natural ingredient resource is the ultimate cure. For many decades, health researchers have been committed to bringing us healthy alternative products to use instead of drugs from pharmaceutical companies.

We can transform our health for the better when we put the proper superfoods and super ingredients into our bodies. Plant-based foods are packed with antioxidants (which remove damaging agents in a living organism), nutrients, and minerals that regulate our pH levels and support every system of the body. This covers everything from mental functioning to the immune system.

## MY COVID-19 VACCINE TRANSFORMATION

I went through a very dark period in life after being forced to get the COVID vaccine. It was a very hard decision; my higher self knew I should not do it.

Many of my friends, my family, and the workforce were pushing the vaccine. Billboards, commercials, bus stop signs, overhead freeway signs pumped us with "Get the vaccine" promotions. I made an appointment to get the vaccine three times and didn't show up. I just knew my DNA didn't need or want it.

I am into holistic health and fitness, I don't drink, and I eat healthy for the most part. But when I caved and got the vaccine, my entire world turned upside down. Over the weeks that followed, I witnessed my body, mind, and soul change from the toxicity that overcame me. My workload had doubled, which caused stress, and I felt completely weighed down with responsibilities. My life force was diminishing as I thought, *Is this really all there is?*

I truly believe the first dose I got was way too much for my small body. I believe I was given the wrong dosage. I weigh 125 pounds. I couldn't understand why I would get the same dose as a man that weighed 250 pounds. I didn't want to get the second dose and called my doctor over Zoom. He proceeded to tell me that I needed to get that second dose. So I reluctantly went in. I resolved to turn on my superpowers to flush it out of my system.

In the months that followed, I shut down, went into a cocoon, and removed myself from society altogether. I stopped communicating with my friends and family and didn't really want to partake in life. I stopped working out, I stopped eating right, and I stopped taking my vitamins and supplements. I went from a self-sufficient, thriving woman to a fragile little girl who wouldn't go out in the sun. I was on the brink of letting go of life.

People around me were saying they experienced no side effects from the vaccine. So how could I express my issues when they had just discredited them? My mother told me stories of people complaining of arthritis, and she said it was all in their heads. I withdrew and went within. My hands had been hurting since the vaccine, but expressing this would only waste more of my precious energy.

A few months later, on another Zoom call with my doctor, he confessed that I was doing so much more for my health than he was. He admitted that I was much more knowledgeable and disciplined on the subjects of foods to eat, exercise, sleep, etc. I realized it was time to switch doctors and always trust my gut.

Then the universe intervened. I was guided to heal from the inside out. I did the research, found the Spring Aqua water, and didn't hesitate to get the system installed. The cost was way more than I wanted to spend, but when it comes to the question of whether you want to be there to raise your kid or not, live or not live, you make different choices. Money suddenly became no object. Good health trumps wealth.

## HEALTH TRANSFORMED

Still desperate to try anything, I kept doing my research to heal my body, mind, and soul, asking tons of questions. My life changed when I met a man named Tig, who was in his late sixties. He literally radiated good health and looked like he was in his fifties. His life force energy was bursting out of him. I said, "What are you doing? I want some of that."

This magic man introduced me to PEMF—pulsated electromagnetic field therapy—and high-grade nutritional supplements. PEMF uses low field magnetic stimulation to heal the body. He had been around the block a few times, and I could tell he knew his stuff. He had tried many products in his lifetime, accomplished many tasks, and carried wisdom that entranced me. We can learn a lot from our elders if we are willing to listen, ask questions, and pay attention.

He introduced me to a healing center where I could try out the PEMF mat and connected me with a nurse who works with cancer patients and is a representative for the nutritional company. The nurse was all about nutrition and healing others, and she put me on a nutritional reset system.

So I went on this amazing healing journey, combining PEMF therapy, nutrition coaching, nutritional supplements, and living water while maintaining my juicing protocol and organic health foods intake. I rid my body of toxins, metals, and stuck energy as I rebuilt and regenerated my body. It helped me build back up the muscle mass I had lost from shutting down and giving up on working out and taking care of myself. The nutrients my body needed so desperately were getting sent to all the right places. I detoxed my system and rebuilt my cellular regeneration capability.

I ended up purchasing the PEMF set with the mat so I could use it on a daily basis to ensure good health alignment. I will share more about this exceptional product later in this book. These mats and devices are a well-kept secret. They are pricey products not covered by health insurance, but the benefits far outweigh the cost. These mats help carry the nutrients and oxygen right into the bloodstream.

As I combined all my resources and became lighter, I noticed a difference in my skin, my aura, and my body and soul. My mind became clear.

I tried these nutritional products for four months before I wrote about it here. I wanted to be able to talk about what all of this did for me. Combining living water, PEMF therapy, and nutritional supplements has given me the lowest blood pressure I have ever had. I lost my belly fat and recently had my heart checked and learned all my arteries are in excellent health. I'm officially off my thyroid medicine after ten years. When I saw my cardiologist, she asked me what I was doing. When I told her, she asked me to drop off information on the Spring Aqua water filtration system.

What I am doing is working. I have seen, felt, and witnessed the results, and they have been documented by my doctor. I have removed a lifetime of toxins from my body by combining all these holistic healing modalities.

. . .

## MAKE IT A LIFESTYLE

I have noticed drastic recent changes in our society. People have become angry, frustrated, easily aggravated, negative, brain fogged, and some are carrying PTSD from all the pandemic chaos. We are all vibrating at very low levels. The goal is to raise our vibration once again.

Friends often call me, asking for help—asking me what I'm doing. I tell them to stop drinking for thirty days, and then we start a customized healing program geared toward the individual. A lot of them are experiencing pain in their third eye and slowed brain activity, in addition to severe heart conditions, which I believe has resulted from the COVID vaccine.

Nutritional products are becoming more popular and important than ever for maintaining our holistic health. Many new products have surfaced, bringing in unusual herbs for healing and made with the most potent superfoods, such a spirulina, wheatgrass, beets, and aloe, and for flushing heavy metals out of the body naturally. Rare mushroom blends are being generated to treat respiratory, immune, and lung function issues; some examples include the agarikon mushroom and lion's mane mushroom for gut, digestive, memory, focus, and clarity benefits. These superfoods supercharge your superpowers. Every nutrient comes right from Mother Nature. They use the purest foods of the highest quality from organic farms around the globe.

You don't have to use the resources I am suggesting. However, I want to show you what worked for me, thereby giving you the option to take control of your own health; please go to my website to learn more: https://www.LuminaryHealingCenter.com. Everything that I have gone through was meant to come to a head here, with me sharing my wisdom to help you transform your mind, body, and soul. We will heal the world together by aligning with the highest vibration we can achieve.

Using living water, PEMF, organic foods, juicing, and nutritional supplements is a lifestyle. So when you make the choice to go all in, be ready to activate your superpowers.

### JOURNAL: Chapter 2

1. What superfoods do our bodies need to thrive?
2. What are the ways we can ensure our bodies get the right nutrients?
3. What foods can you cut out? What foods can you add to your diet?

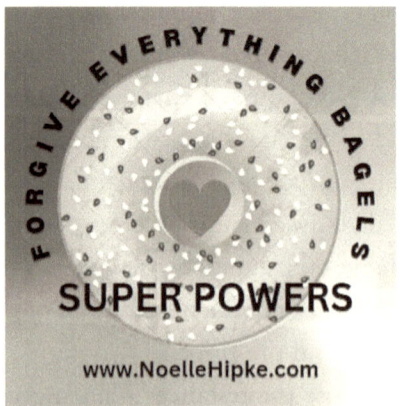

## CHAPTER THREE

# IDENTITY

They say you don't become a mature adult until you are fifty. With a higher perspective earned over a lifetime, you gain understanding of how things are done. I am writing this book now to empower you with wisdom and knowledge at a younger age. If you internalize this incredible information and data, you will transcend to a higher level. I call this leveling up.

When you level up, sometimes you outgrow the people around you. You might not relate to friends—and sometimes family members—as you previously used to. From birth, our belief systems have been formed by what other people want and expect from us. Now is the time to change that. This is the new earth where you become who you are meant to be, not what anybody else wants you to be. You can figure out who you are by analyzing your DNA and following your heart-and-soul guidance; what feels right to you is what is right for you. Do not let other people dictate who you are.

We can spend all our lives trying to please other people, and we may never succeed. The only person you need to please is yourself. In order to do that, you have to shut out the chatter of the world, friends, coworkers, and sometimes your parents. If they are already set in their ways, there might be no changing that.

I am going to cover a lot of topics in this section. You may very well have faced some of these uncomfortable circumstances. My goal is to help you identify patterns, sequences, belief systems, behavior, etc., so we can put an end to the negative cycles.

# SCHOOL

## Elementary School

Elementary school is by far the freest time of your academic life. All you have to do is be a kid, run on the playground, and learn the basics of life. At least, this was the way it was in the 1970s. We had dodgeball, kickball, foursquare, wall ball, the jungle gym, and monkey bars. It was heaven.

However, school has changed in the era of cell phones and the internet. Kids are growing up faster than they used to. We have all these new distractions. As parents, we need to pay attention to what information is going into our kids' heads; this is going to shape how they think and act and what they will become and believe in the future. We must spend more time educating our kids, paying attention, and talking about things we didn't expect to at such a young age. No topic should be off limits. If we don't teach them, someone else will. Do we want someone else's beliefs imprinting on our kids? Or do we want to empower our kids with the knowledge we have gained and help them make better choices and know what to expect?

Also, the expectations for young kids today are much higher; the pressure to learn basic mathematics, science, etc., has created GATE programs, also known as gifted children's programs and high school levels in some systems.

## Junior High School

One of the biggest transitions in life is going into junior high school. Different elementary schools meld together to form the new class, and now you are not learning in one classroom but in many different classrooms and from many different teachers. Friends divide, and new groups are formed: jocks, band geeks, cheerleaders, dorks, intellectuals, etc. You are suddenly judged based on your clothes, how you look, what you own, and what your parents own. Everyone is labeled. Yuck.

Back in the 1970s and 1980s, usually the mother stayed home to raise the kids while dad went to work. In our family, my mother sewed our clothes, cleaned the home, did the cooking, and reared the kids, while dad worked a full-time job, maintained the yard, washed the cars, and made repairs on the home. Due to only one working parent, money was tight, and multiple traits and skills were required in order to maintain life and a household. We learned to be happy off very little income and live a simple life.

Times have really changed, with both parents often working these days just to stay afloat. Now everyone is busy spending time and energy in other areas of life due to the internet, while many of the simplicities of life have been dismissed.

## High School

I am not going to lie: high school is one of the most uncomfortable times in life. People are mean, hurtful, judgmental, aggressive, ruthless, bullying, opinionated, disrespectful, hormonal, moody, and dealing with lots of changes and challenges. And today the pressure and stress to perform at top levels is even more compounded. Social value is defined by what phone/computer/gizmos you have, your shoes/clothes, handbags, sunglasses, and of course the type of vehicle you drive.

• • •

# MATERIALISM: HOUSEWIVES OF HUNTINGTON BEACH

Your identity forms throughout your life. You have the power to change it and reinvent yourself at any time. I have learned never to say never; when I learn a lesson, often my viewpoint changes, and I do the exact thing I said I would never do.

When I was a teenager driving to school one day, I glanced up at a woman in a beautiful, brand-new, white SUV. She looked like she had it all: a gorgeous wedding ring on her finger, manicured nails, light-blond hair, designer sunglasses, and two beautiful young children in the back of the car. I thought she must have the perfect life. I wanted that.

In time, I eventually did earn that, but I had to encounter a lot of things along the way to get there. And when I got there, it wasn't always as good as I thought it would be.

I'm going to jump ahead to when I was married and my son was around seven or eight, in 2007. This was the moment in my life when I knew I had it all. I had hit my magic moment of achieving the ultimate dream. We were sitting at a friend's house in their beautifully manicured backyard, watching our kids swim in their rock-style pool. Our husbands were barbecuing while we sat in lounge chairs, sipping wine, listening to music, nibbling on appetizers. Sounds lovely, right? For a few summers, I would sit there thinking, *This is the perfect life*. If I could freeze time and go back to any moment, this is definitely the moment I would pick.

Our group began to grow as we connected with other families in the area through the sports our kids played, so parties and gatherings often included multiple families and kids, with boys and girls interacting. Many of us mothers didn't work full-time. I worked part-time, balancing being a working mom and a stay-at-home at the same time. The idea was to be able to bring in some income in addition to being there to drive our kids to after-school sports and help with homework and doctor appointments.

At one point, I realized I was hanging out with the housewives of Huntington Beach. Now, reality shows were just surfacing, and there wasn't one for moms of Huntington Beach, but I often felt like I was in the middle of my own TV scene without the film crew. Materialistic things became really important. It was a big deal if someone in the group got a new car. Then it became the clothes, like a new style of jeans someone bought: everybody had to go out and get that $150 pair of jeans. If a girl got a new handbag, we oohed and aahed over it. Remodeling the home, redecorating, jewelry, etc.—it was all about who had what, who could afford what, and who bought what.

It was meaningless.

I was already working as a Realtor with a special focus on the elderly. The elderly are frequently taken advantage of and abused due to their diminished capacity from medications, lack of nutrition, or being otherwise impaired. I focused on helping seniors with Alzheimer's who were entering retirement and assisted-living communities. I saw what grown children went through to make sure their aging parents were taken care of accordingly. And the price tag was not cheap. Do you know in 2022 it could cost close to $10,000 per month to have your parent in an assisted-living community with special accommodations? I saw entire families ripped apart from the decisions people had to make under stressful circumstances no one had ever prepared them for. At the same time, I witnessed my fellow housewives spend that amount on a whim.

I also saw homes filled to the brim with crap that family members were responsible for cleaning and clearing out, often burdening people who lived in other states with the responsibility of traveling to address the monumental issue as well as to sell the home.

As you get older, you realize the stuff you've gathered doesn't mean anything. Yep, I said that. What matters is how you feel and prosper energetically, mentally, physically, emotionally, and spiritually in your lifetime.

• • •

## THE MIND

Here I am going to introduce you to how the mind works before delving into behaviors to keep an eye out for.

The mind allows you to be aware of the environment and your experiences—to feel, to think, to function in the world. This makes up a person's intellect. The mind dictates imagination, memory, sensations, thought, and will. The mind reasons, perceives, comprehends, thinks, and functions.

## The Conscious and Unconscious Mind

The conscious mind holds memories, feelings, and thoughts we are aware of. It functions as short-term memory, and its capacity is limited. Your consciousness consists of your self-awareness and awareness of the world around you.

The subconscious mind is not immediately accessible to consciousness and comprises our memories, values, and beliefs and monitors information around us. It affects our feelings and behaviors without awareness. It processes and stores information to use at a later date.

## Subliminal Messages

Subliminal messages arrive below the baseline of consciousness or feeling sensations—ideas that may be remembered due to constant repetition but are not perceived or recognized and can therefore influence the mind without our being aware of it.

This is why you see the same advertisements over and over. Advertisers are trying to get you to think about the product without your even realizing it. They want you to buy it, even if you don't need it or want it. Subliminal messages can also be used to make you think and feel a certain way, like that you need to look skinnier, younger, smarter, prettier, buffer, and the list goes on. This technique has been used for decades on TV commercials but has gotten way out of hand due to the proliferation of the internet and cell phones. And now advertisers can track your searches, conversations, and even your brain patterns to manipulate what you think, feel, and do.

Now, that is some pretty wild stuff. Being aware of this phenomenon is the only way to learn to control what you expose yourself to. This is why turning off your devices for days at a time could do wonders for your health.

Let me tell you a secret that I will probably mention several times because it's that important: I haven't watched the news in over twenty years. Yes, I said that. And you know what? I am the happiest I have ever been. I can't do anything about what is happening in the world in the moment. I can't control it, and I can't change it, but I can feel it. And if I watched it, I'd dream about it. Yuck. At one time I considered becoming an anchorwoman; then I realized that the news almost never reports on good stories, only bad stories. Who wants that negativity in their brain? I shut the news off altogether and never looked back.

Don't worry. Enough people around you will watch the news and feel the need to report it to you, and you will find you aren't missing much. However, you will feel their stressed-out energy when they share the data they have been exposed to, reminding you that you are better off not bothering with it.

The internet, social media, and news channels influence how we make our decisions. If the news tells you home buyers aren't buying homes, people stop buying homes, and voilà, a trend is started. The news cycle affects the economy and is a great way to manipulate the masses into performing in conscious, subconscious, unconscious behavior patterns. Get enough people thinking, believing, and behaving a certain way, and you push the vibrational energetic frequency of an entire collective group in the same direction. This creates a massive movement in support of a given agenda, positive or negative; think of it like a crowd in a sports stadium doing the wave. So you can't believe all the mainstream media, as well as everything you read and see online and hear on radio and televisions stations, because it is riddled with information meant to control the population. Publications might be trying to persuade you to believe things that simply are not true—all to raise the number of viewers and clicks on links to news stories.

Now, if we could get everyone on the planet to pay attention to changing their behaviors for the better, reprogramming themselves to a positive mindset, and moving in the right direction to heal themselves, they will naturally heal each other, and that is when we create heaven on the new earth.

I once worked with a man in his early fifties who was very sick and going through dialysis (dialysis is when you receive blood transfusions through an IV needle to try and clean the blood in your body; it's uncomfortable and usually very painful). When we discussed business on the phone, I would hear the TV news on full blast in the background. I discovered some people like to have the news on in the background when they are at home or falling asleep.

Do not do this or make this a habit. It is bad for you. I asked him if he had the TV news on all the time, and he confirmed. Think about it. He absorbs it auditorily *and* visually—a double whammy to the brain. No wonder he was so sick.

## Unconscious Mind

The unconscious mind is not accessible to the conscious mind. It impacts our behavior and emotions without our awareness. It is basically anything going on in the body that we are not paying attention to. When in this state of mind, we lack awareness and perception. This in turn can make you nonreactive to stimulations you need to react to.

Okay, here I am going to delve into drugs and alcohol. When you put drugs and alcohol into your body, your unconscious and subconscious mind take over, tossing out your conscious mind. Your conscious mind helps you make good choices. But when your unconscious and subconscious minds take over, you are giving your power away. In order to stay in your superpowers, you need to be clear, intentional, aware, and direct.

Many people turn to drugs and alcohol to numb their feelings. This brings on a slew of problems: emotions run high, and you alternately feel numb, fearless, free, etc. You often don't remember what you did, how you got somewhere, or what you said. This can get you into a whole lot of trouble. When intoxicated, we might think we are letting go of it all when in actuality we are pushing our emotions down to avoid dealing with the true issue at hand.

When you are going through a very hard time, you are being called to level up, address the situation head-on, feel it, and move through it. You must sail right into the storm of transition. Transition can be very uncomfortable. You are changing your DNA, your lineage, your beliefs, your rights, and learning what is right and correct for *you*.

Your entire life is about finding your power and energy within. People will try to take, control, and manipulate your power. It is up to you to control who has access to it, who you will share it with, and what you will ultimately do with it.

• • •

## IDENTIFYING NEGATIVE BEHAVIORS

I am going to identify here negative behaviors that you are most likely to face in your lifetime. Many people turn to these negative behaviors because that is what was modeled to them—by their parents and grandparents, for example, and by the generations before them. It may also be genetically imbedded in their DNA. We are going to address these items so you can use your superpowers and knowledge to change the course of history.

The real power here is being able to forgive people for their choices and behaviors; many times, they don't even realize what they are doing due to the subconscious and unconscious mind having taken over, which we will address here as well. Many people turn to drugs, alcohol, gambling, and other addictions when they have not dealt with their own emotions and issues. I will provide ideas on how to handle and heal those issues on your own so you can put solutions into place and are not facing the struggle alone. By activating your superpowers, you will know how to figure it out and level up.

## Alcoholism

My dad was an alcoholic, his father was an alcoholic, and my stepfather was an alcoholic. I have grown up and been exposed to a rather toxic environment all my life. That is what has been modeled for me. When you are in this type of environment at a young age, you learn techniques to get you through it. Back in the day, I had no choices. But today, I will provide you the knowledge so you can use your superpowers to do what you need to do for you.

If your parents and family drink and your household feels uncomfortable and you feel like you are walking on eggshells, hiding to avoid being hurt, and avoiding home, seek out a counselor or mentor. Alcoholics often abuse those around them—mentally, physically, emotionally, energetically, and spiritually. We need to get you help so you can understand and process the situation in order to stop this pattern; otherwise, you are stuck in a cycle that can pass down from generation to generation, and it will affect you consciously and unconsciously for the rest of your life.

I started taking care of myself at fourteen. I never knew what mood my parents would be in, and my environment always felt unstable. Alcoholism makes people volatile, toxic, aggressive, angry, moody, unpredictable. Sounds crazy, right? Yet they will make you think and feel like you are the crazy one.

In junior high, my stepdad forced me to become Catholic. A lot of parents want to look to outsiders like they are doing the right thing while modeling a totally different behavior behind closed doors. If I didn't get up and go to church, my parents took away my phone, my TV, and put me on restriction. So I was forced to do something I didn't want to do by a man who mistreated me. My stepfather had never had kids of his own; he took on a wife with three kids he didn't know how to raise and pretty much modeled the behavior that was taught to him.

My stepfather demanded we do household chores, which is perfectly normal. However, at the age of seventeen, I was working part-time at Medieval Times as a photo wench in order to pay my tuition for my senior year at a private high school, so I tended to work late nights. My stepdad expected us to get up bright and early on Saturday mornings to cheerfully do household chores. Obviously, my body was still growing, and I usually got very little sleep before he marched in my room between 7 and 8 a.m., demanding that I get up.

Groggy, tired, and not at all responding to the way this man was treating me, I would ignore him and roll over as he yelled in my face. He would get so worked up that he would spit all over me. When I refused to acknowledge his bad behavior, he would get a bucket of cold water and douse me with it in my bed. Now I could no longer ignore the uncomfortable situation he had placed me in. I would drag myself out of bed and be forced to do chores like using a toothbrush to clean the grout between the tiles in the walkway. The man had abnormal anger issues, and his way of trying to control me was very unhealthy. I often left my house to run around my neighborhood as fast as I could, tears streaming down my face. I ran and cried until I could not stand up anymore. I didn't know what else to do; my body's instinct was to push out and release the toxic energy.

If you are not careful, you will repeat the patterns that were modeled for you. After work, I would hang out with coworkers ten years older than me, drinking and partying to stay away from my household. You might think this kind of activity is fun, but it damages your body and mind and sets you up for poor judgment and scary scenarios you would never wish upon anyone. You just don't realize it at the time—because you feel numb and don't care.

We are not taught how to be parents. We are students all our lives. The only thing we can do is be aware of the cycle and learn how to break and change it.

Many of you may face toxic situations. I want you to know that the best way to heal and move on with your life is to forgive anyone and everyone who has ever hurt you. Yes, I am talking about the girls and guys who have mistreated you, or a family member who has abused you. This is the only way to heal and move forward in a healthy way. The issue was with them, not you.

Forgiveness is an internal exercise, so yes, it can be granted from a distance anytime and doesn't have to be face-to-face. Listen to meditations on forgiveness. Forgive yourself for "allowing" it to happen (you will likely blame yourself even though you shouldn't), and forgive them.

By forgiving, you allow your body to heal and release the trauma, which in turn prevents the illness derived from keeping it trapped in the body.

Check out the book *12 Steps on Buddha's Path* by Laura S. for an alternative to the traditional Alcoholic Anonymous books on the shelf.

## Drugs

Drugs can take over your life and make you someone else. They hijack your body and prevent you from thinking, feeling, and experiencing clearly, and you completely lose all of your superpowers. You are cut off at the knees from reaching your full potential. Drugs are evil.

When you take drugs, you open the door for bad things to happen to you and to surround and encompass you. It is one of the most unwise choices you can make. Others will pressure you because they have their own agenda. They either want to make money off selling them to you, bring you down, see you fail, control you, or hurt you. They do not have your best interests in mind. When kids say drugs are cool, they are the fools. Never have I heard of someone being successful and at the top of their game when they were on drugs. Athletes are disqualified if they show signs of drug use. You don't need drugs at all when you are aligned with your superpowers.

My son went to Huntington High, which was nicknamed Heroin High due to the immense drug problem in the school system. Orange County was becoming the hot spot for kids overdosing on drugs because of easy access to their parents' medicine cabinets. Drug abuse quickly took over these kids' lives, often claiming them forever.

My friends who had a teenage boy struggled greatly. Their son was breaking into cars at night, stealing anything he could sell for more drugs. His behavior wreaked havoc on their family and sanity. He got caught and arrested, and his mother was given the option to spend $35,000 to send him to a drug rehabilitation center in the middle of nowhere. She was tight on money and wasn't sure if it was worth the funds. I told her, "If you don't send him and he overdoses and dies, you are going to beat yourself up for the rest of your life for not sending him to that center."

Kids can have a very hard life if they get mixed up with the wrong people and make the wrong choices. Drugs can mess you up forever. Avoid this path at all costs, and stay away from people who try to take you down with them.

Alcohol and drugs turn you into a robot. Simple as that.

The documentary film *Overtaken* was released in 2012 when kids were dying from overdoses left and right. When I saw the film, I knew I had to share it with others, and I brought it to our local school district. You can currently find the film on YouTube. And I highly suggest kids and parents watch it together and talk about it. This is a very real thing that we need to address.

## Marijuana/Ganja/Pot

I smoked marijuana for twenty-six years, even when it wasn't legal. And I missed out on half my life because I was numb, unaware, and untapped into the world and the people around me. If you are an empath, you may discover the urge to turn to drugs and alcohol. Empaths see, feel, and witness life on a deeper and different level than most, so they tend to look for an outlet to dull their senses.

If you notice you enjoy your alone time and prefer to stay away from certain situations and people, you could very well be an empath. Books such as *The Empath's Survival Guide* by Judith Orloff might be helpful; there are other books on empaths as well. As we transcend and become more aware and activate our superpowers, our senses become more enhanced. So be prepared to feel more, experience more, and understand more than you ever have.

Get ready for this next segment.

What happens to the human body when you smoke marijuana? You dull your senses and awareness of what is happening around you and to you. Marijuana consumes your superpowers, sending you into a low vibration, which allows the energy from your devices to tap into your brain.

When you are high and go online, subliminal messages enter your subconscious and unconscious mind, possibly brainwashing you to believe, think, and feel things that are not real. Think a virtual reality takeover in your brain. When you are tapped into your superpowers, you realize what you are here to do and automatically disconnect from negative situations. The only way to stay tapped in is to clean your system and body of all toxins. Stay free and clear of drugs, booze, and medications (when possible) at all costs. You will gain clarity and control of your destiny.

In this day and age, pot is both legal and way more potent than it used to be. The THC levels are so dang high, which causes anxiety and affects our central nervous systems. When you think you are calming your body, there is a very good chance you will experience the opposite effect—only you don't know that because you are led to believe it helps you.

When I removed the toxicity of marijuana from my body, the knowledge, wisdom, and clarity that poured into me was beyond anything I could have imagined. I understood things that the normal person cannot explain or comprehend, creating a magnificent, powerful, universal life force energy flow. You can tap right into your own source of energy.

• • •

## TYPES OF ABUSE

There are many types of abuse. When I was a kid, I swore to myself I would never stay in an abusive relationship. I didn't know at the time that there are many kinds of abuse, some of which are invisible and hard to identify. But as I grew older and acquired wisdom, experience, and knowledge, I learned how to spot it.

Often, we get a feeling in our bodies before we achieve conscious awareness. That is called our intuition or instinct. Or bodies are magnificent, reliable sources that tell us what is right for us and not right for us. Tuning in and listening to yourself is the key to keeping your superpowers turned on.

## Physical

I used to think that physical abuse was the only type of abuse because it is the only kind that leaves physical evidence, such as a black eye or a broken arm. Physical abuse comprises both mental abuse and emotional abuse; what someone does to you physically also affects you emotionally and mentally, ultimately shaping how you will react and make decisions for the rest of your life. Physical abuse occurs when someone hits you or hurts you with an object such as their hand, a belt, or wooden spoon. Back in my day, people would take a belt to their kids as punishment. This torture goes way back in history, to the whipping of slaves. So when I say these patterns and traits have been carried down for generations, I mean it. These patterns and traits are often in our DNA, waiting to be triggered when something activates our flight-or-fight response.

## Mental

Mental abuse is a form of manipulation and control that often involves distorting someone's sense of reality. The effects of mental abuse are just as detrimental as those of physical abuse. You will find this type of abuse in households, at work, and at school, used by people who want you to perform, think, or be a certain way.

Examples: threats of violence or abandonment, intentionally frightening someone, making an individual fear that they will not receive the food or care they need, lying, making derogatory or slanderous statements about an individual to others.

## Emotional

Emotional abuse is closely linked to mental abuse and can happen to anyone at any time in their lives. Children, teens, and adults all experience emotional abuse at some point or another. It is meant to undermine your self-esteem and make you feel worse about yourself and can have devastating consequences on all involved and affect a lifetime of relationships. Just because there is no physical mark doesn't mean the abuse isn't real.

Emotional abuse derives from any act pursuing confinement, isolation, humiliation, intimidation, verbal assaults, or behaviors that deplete one's sense of dignity, self-worth, and identity. People who have been subjected to emotional abuse tend to display personality changes and low self-esteem and become withdrawn, depressed, anxious, or suicidal.

Emotional abuse can also include withholding important documentation or information, demeaning an individual because of their nationality or the language they speak, intentionally misinterpreting traditional practices, making someone feel they are too much trouble, excessively criticizing, being disrespectful, ordering an individual around unreasonably, or treating an individual like a servant or child.

Emotional abuse, like other types of abuse, tends to take the form of a generational cycle. In relationships, this cycle starts when one partner emotionally abuses the other, typically to show control and dominance. The consequences of the abuser's performance generates guilt, and then the abuser makes up excuses for their own behavior to avoid taking responsibility. The abuser proceeds to behave as if the abuse never occurred and may turn on charm by becoming giving and apologetic, which in turn makes the abused party believe the abuser is sorry or that they haven't been truly abused.

## Spiritual and Religious

I do believe there is such a thing as spiritual abuse. I would even consider calling it soul abuse. People are attacking your spirit and soul when they hurt you mentally, emotionally, physically, verbally, and energetically. Some people harness belief systems as a way to control and manipulate others—to make people feel bad about themselves; to control how they act; to condemn them for not doing things, being things, and believing things others deem necessary. Religious beliefs do not make it okay to force, manipulate, reject, torture, control, judge, ridicule, hurt, compare, restrict, ignore, disrespect, punish, or exterminate someone for having a difference of opinion. Isn't religion about accepting and loving all types of people, no matter their differences, all pointing to the same concept of one source?

Now, I am not a big fan of talking about hot button issues, but I have to address my experience on this topic so you can understand. I have been exposed to many religions in my lifetime: Catholicism, Christianity, Buddhism, Scientology, and Judaism. I was forced to become Catholic, my ex-husband was an avid Christian, and my sister ventured into Scientology.

I would like to address Scientology because I just got hit with it hard while meditating today. I never got involved with the Church of Scientology personally. However, I like to keep a very open mind, and today I read the energy of this religion. And the message I got from my observation is this:

- Twenty-five years ago, Scientology was ahead of its time and misunderstood.
- People dismissed Scientology, claiming it was not a religion.
- People judged this religion based on its unusual principles regarding working with science.
- Scientology was all about deprogramming and reprogramming the mind using science, hence the name *Scien*tology.

Scientology basically involves clearing out your childhood trauma, cleaning up your DNA, and surrounding yourself with like-minded individuals in order to thrive. Other people's belief systems and those people triggering us keep us stuck. Scientology works hard to remove people from toxic situations and from their families to help the individual gain control and reprogram their mind. This is probably why Scientology has been discredited as a cult. In order to change the negatively programmed, generational home pattern, Scientologists must be dislodged, reprogramed, and helped to realign with society. This process takes time, commitment, and money, hence why monetary donations are emphasized.

I remember my sister doing deep cleanses by sitting in a sauna for possibly seven hours a day for several days in a row. She was detoxing everything from her body, mind, and soul—from dental injections to tooth repair to antibiotics she took as a kid. And when you go into these deep states of repair, you go into deep meditations and deep surrenders. You start to see things clearly. And when you can see things clearly, you are able to forgive and understand why people do the things you normally can't understand.

People often judge what they don't understand as batshit crazy. You change your vibration when you detox, allowing you to see things from multiple perspectives. Scientology basically creates a new person. When I look back, I see that my sister thrived from this advanced programming. She became ultra-successful once she was able to hone and own her life. Embracing her uniqueness, she stepped into her superpowers without letting anyone else determine who she was. She wore Scientology jewelry and stood her ground and leveled up over and over.

As a single woman, she owned her own five-bedroom house in Los Angeles, California, and was VP of client relations at an engineering and construction firm that couldn't live without her. She didn't have children, which allowed her to neither trigger DNA or childhood issues from raising children nor pass down any abuse patterns. She thrived on all levels because she was only responsible for herself, her pets, and her belongings.

Another issue I want to bring up here is that the Scientologist L. Ron Hubbard was working with life force energy in each being, healing childhood trauma and redirecting it. He also believed in UFOs and extraterrestrials, something many people didn't and still don't believe in, which discredited his works. However, as I've gotten older and more experienced, I see a very distinct possibility that we are all from different planets in different galaxies. Many differences, energies, frequencies, and cultures exist here on this planet, and each person's DNA is unique. And now we have cross-pollinated and shared our DNA with many other races, hence the ability to either become one or turn to hate. Right now, we are in recalibration and realignment—right in the middle of a transition.

## Extraterrestrials (ETs) and Entities

This seems like a perfect time to move into this topic. I have to admit, I used to think people who believe in UFOs and ETs were a bit "off." However, since becoming single at the age of forty-five, I have had five different men tell me they know they are species from other planets and galaxies. They know exactly where they are from and what they represent, and they have ideas and concepts the typical person could never imagine.

At first I thought, *Okay, guy; you are out there.* Now I see it differently. You can only see it for yourself when you are hit with the information in just the right way at the right time. These men were older and had been studying history, ancient civilizations, and visiting sacred sites to connect. I now realize they were likely single because they were selective with what species they allowed into their biofield.

I wasn't sure if I should share this information; I know it's out there. But go outside and look at the sky. See the entire universe that we have been ignoring for far too long. Have you ever wondered what might exist beyond Earth? If aliens have spaceships, that means their technology is way more advanced than ours. Heck, half of the world could be equipped with artificially intelligent, human-looking clones and we might not know the difference. We are definitely coming into the age of technology and a massive shift in evolution. So, if you want to think I am a little off, I am so okay with that. I am not going to apologize for the things I feel, understand, and see that others cannot. I am just here to share the knowledge and break it to you gently.

I have connected the dots between a lot of data from around 200 references, which are included in the back of this book for you to research, and have combined that data with my personal experiences in order to generate these viewpoints.

What are entities? Entities comprise invisible energy that exists apart from the physical plane. They are operating in a higher density we cannot see or feel, in the third dimension. Nevertheless, they hijack and impact, positively or negatively, many human beings and behaviors without our permission or knowledge. The lower your vibration, the easier it is for entities to hijack the body and overtake your personality, decision-making abilities, and daily reasoning—hence the need to understand that many humans are not operating at full capacity one hundred percent of the time. The paranormal and ghosts also fall into this category.

Some ET species and entities attack energetically, disabling other species mentally, emotionally, and physically. This is done through manipulation, lies, deceit, abuse, booze and drugs, the digital matrix, electronic devices, worldwide online group events, rape, human trafficking, social media, and press. Think about it. When an ET or entity attacks or abducts someone, that individual is often unable to function properly, causing paralysis, PTSD, mental anguish, changes in behavior, sleep deprivation, loss of focus, brain fog, and other things of this nature.

What do these ETs and entities want from you? Your life force energy. I will cover more about this in the next chapter. Who wouldn't want to use energy for their own benefit? We can do so on a daily basis when we are in tune and using it intentionally. The ones who are intentional are working with energy, telepathy, meditation, nature, clairvoyance, clairaudience, clairsentience, clairalience, clairgustance.

One man told me he saw UFOs above a volcano he had been hiking up and got lost on for hours. He remembers it being freezing cold. Another man used a meditation technique that allowed him ascension travel. In my dreams, I have gone to other planets, been in several spaceships, and have had my body affected by ETs. More and more people these days are being affected by ETs and entities and are being triggered to wake up. It is time for us to ascend and evolve together. So, kids, you are going to be the first generation exposed to the truth. ETs are real, and they are here on earth, walking among us; there is a chance you might be one of them. And this might be a hard one to swallow, but it can be a beautiful one as well. You are the chosen ones to evolve this planet to a higher frequency. Before you came down to earth, you knew you were going to be assigned the monumental task to help humanity heal, and you took it on, willingly and knowingly. You are the ones who will create an evolutionary change in the entire universe.

Now, that is some pretty profound information. It is literally giving my body the tingles as I write this. I didn't expect to talk about this, but I am being compelled to. Either step into your powers for the good of humanity, or destroy the earth and each other. Which one will you choose? And I want you to consider the following questions: What if? Then what? Now what?

Consider Earth as the hub of many types of species from different planets in different galaxies, each species with its own superpowers, hence the reason we are all different. We have chosen to come down here to connect, evolve, align, harmonize, learn from one another, and see if we can carry out our soul destiny. I believe when you address your karmic lessons, heal your soul, and carry out your soul destiny, you move up to an elevated level and do not return to this planet. How do I know this? I just know it in my bones.

On a related note: one day, a woman healer picked me out of the crowd, walked up to me, and said, "Do you know this is your last time on Planet Earth?"

I looked at her directly in the eye with a straight face and said,

"Would you believe me if I told you yes?"

Synchronicity confirmation granted. Thank you, universe!

## Sexual Abuse

Sexual abuse is unwanted sexual activity where perpetrators use force, make threats, or take advantage of victims who are unable to give consent. An American is sexually assaulted every sixty-eight seconds. Most victims and perpetrators know each other. Immediate reactions to sexual abuse include shock, fear, or disbelief. Long-term symptoms include anxiety, fear, or post-traumatic stress disorder.

These following sexual violence statistics are from a few years back. However, the numbers are still shocking, which is why I choose to include them as a reference. It doesn't matter what year it is. This behavior is unacceptable and off the charts.

The following statistics are quoted directly from https://www.rainn.org/statistics/victims-sexual-violence.

- On average, there are 463,634 victims (age 12 or older) of rape and sexual assault each year in the United States.

### Younger People Are at the Highest Risk of Sexual Violence

- Ages 12-34 are the highest risk years for rape and sexual assault.
- Those age 65 and older are 92% less likely than 12-24 year olds to be a victim of rape or sexual assault, and 83% less likely than 25-49 year olds.

### Women and Girls Experience Sexual Violence at High Rates

Millions of women in the United States have experienced rape.

- As of 1998, an estimated 17.7 million American women had been victims of attempted or completed rape.

Young women are especially at risk.

- 82% of all juvenile victims are female. 90% of adult rape victims are female.
- Females ages 16-19 are 4 times more likely than the general population to be victims of rape, attempted rape, or sexual assault.
- Women ages 18-24 who are college students are 3 times more likely than women in general to experience sexual violence. Females of the same age who are not enrolled in college are 4 times more likely.

## Men and Boys Are Also Affected by Sexual Violence

Millions of men in the United States have been victims of rape.

- As of 1998, 2.78 million men in the US had been victims of attempted or completed rape.
- About 3% of American men—or 1 in 33—have experienced an attempted or completed rape in their lifetime.
- 1 out of every 10 rape victims are male.

## Sexual Violence Can Have Long-Term Effects on Victims

The likelihood that a person suffers suicidal or depressive thoughts increases after sexual violence.

- 94% of women who are raped experience symptoms of post-traumatic stress disorder (PTSD) during the two weeks following the rape.
- 30% of women report symptoms of PTSD 9 months after the rape.
- 33% of women who are raped contemplate suicide.

- 13% of women who are raped attempt suicide.
- Approximately 70% of rape or sexual assault victims experience moderate to severe distress, a larger percentage than for any other violent crime.

People who have been sexually assaulted are more likely to use drugs than the general public.

- 3.4 times more likely to use marijuana
- 6 times more likely to use cocaine
- 10 times more likely to use other major drugs

Sexual violence also affects victims' relationships with their family, friends, and co-workers.

- 38% of victims of sexual violence experience work or school problems, which can include significant problems with a boss, coworker, or peer.
- 37% experience family/friend problems, including getting into arguments more frequently than before, not feeling able to trust their family/friends, or not feeling as close to them as before the crime.
- 84% of survivors who were victimized by an intimate partner experience professional or emotional issues, including moderate to severe distress, or increased problems at work or school.
- 67% of survivors who were victimized by a stranger experience professional or emotional issues, including moderate to severe distress or increased problems at work or school.

Victims are at risk of pregnancy and sexually transmitted infections or diseases (STIs or STDs).

> ... The average number of rapes and sexual assaults against females of childbearing age is approximately 250,000. Thus, the number of children conceived from rape each year in the

United States might range from 7,750—12,500. This is a very general estimate. . . .

### Native Americans Are at the Greatest Risk of Sexual Violence

On average, American Indians ages 12 and older experience 5,900 sexual assaults per year.

- American Indians are twice as likely to experience a rape/sexual assault compared to all races.
- 41% of sexual assaults against American Indians are committed by a stranger; 34% by an acquaintance; and 25% by an intimate or family member.

### Sexual Violence Affects Thousands of Prisoners Across the Country

An estimated 80,600 inmates each year experience sexual violence while in prison or jail.

- 60% of all sexual violence against inmates is perpetrated by jail or prison staff.
- More than 50% of the sexual contact between inmate and staff member—all of which is illegal—is nonconsensual.

### Sexual Violence in the Military Often Goes Unreported

6,053 military members reported experiencing sexual assault during military service in FY 2018. DoD estimates about 20,500 service members experienced sexual assault that year.

- DoD estimates 6.2% of active duty women and 0.7% of active duty men experienced sexual assault in FY 2018.

## Sexual Assault

I have tried to write this book with personal perspectives as well as factual information. With that in mind, these are my thoughts and beliefs on sex and rape:

1. If you are a pretty girl, you have a very good chance of being plucked from the crowd; think before you drink, do not go anywhere alone with someone you don't know, and don't assume the best of people; predators play into your innocence.

2. Situations where you are not thinking clearly, are not aware of your surroundings, or are with people you don't know and trust should be avoided. Assume everyone is stranger danger until you have spent much more time with them than a few fun hours.

3. Perpetrators might slip a rape drug into your cocktail or drink. You will notice a change in your behavior, the way you feel. You may feel sleepy, dreamy, or out of it and may have a metallic taste in your mouth the next day. Your friends might observe a difference in your behavior, but they might be drinking too, or drugged as well. Always guard your drinks and purses. Never leave them unattended when you hit the dance floor. This gives people the perfect opportunity to drug you or slip a device in your purse to follow you. Even if your friend is watching your drinks and purses, there is no guarantee she will spot danger in a dark club when a cute guy is trying to grab her attention.

4. Do not split up with your friends. If you meet someone, do not go home with them and do not take them to your house. I know people want to hook up and have fun. But honestly, this behavior is just asking for trouble. If someone is interested in you, do not give your power away. Make them earn you, respect you, and prove to you they are worthy of your energy and time. If they are really interested in you, they will ask for

your number and make a true connection by taking the time to get to know you. Ladies, do not offer up sex just to claim someone's time and attention for a few moments. You will feel used and might contract a sexually transmitted disease. Some diseases you carry with you for the rest of your life, such as herpes. It is not worth it.

5. If a guy is willing to hook up with you easily, chances are he has done this with many other women. He is much more susceptible to carrying sexually transmitted diseases (STDs). Did you know some STDs can prevent you from having children in the future if they go undetected? You should require an STD blood test prior to having intercourse with anyone. When dating, I tell men right off the bat that I require an STD test before we get involved sexually. This way, I set the bar and weed out any men who only have an interest in hooking up. Some say their wife had an STD but they didn't, or that their results came back inconclusive; or they disappear. Do yourself a favor and make this a lifelong goal to remove this unnecessary stress and pain.

6. Having sex with anyone and everyone is not good for you. The energy (and DNA) from that person—and the energy (and DNA) from all the people that person has had sex with—goes right into you. Be very picky with who you share energy with. It truly can affect your health, emotions, and overall well-being. A man willing to sleep with you immediately would probably have sex with a call girl or hooker.

7. Giving oral sex can give you an STD. When the semen enters your mouth, it goes right into your bloodstream. Only a guy who loves you and whom you are in love with really deserves that blow job—and he better be willing to get STD tested and reciprocate as well. Even then, that man may cheat on you with another girl, which subjects you to any diseases she may

be carrying. I have heard stories where men have cheated on their wives and given them herpes. Herpes is a lifelong STD you cannot get rid of. It creates visible sores when there is a breakout. However, even if there is no breakout, the STD still exists and can be transferred. I suggest you also get yourself and your partner tested for STDs during your relationship and after a breakup to stay on top of your health.

8. Drinking, doing drugs, and going places with people you don't know create the optimal situations for someone to take advantage of you. Being out and about late at night is incredibly dangerous. I remember walking home in the early-morning hours when the sun was about to come up, and a van full of rowdy, drunk young men drove by. Intuition told me to dive into the bushes, and sure enough that van drove around the block a few times with those boys looking for me, calling out.

   Do not park next to vans or travel alone at night without paying attention to your surroundings. Stay off your phone and arm yourself with mace or some type of protection. Do not walk to your car alone in the dark. Ask someone you know to walk you, and then you can drive them to their car, or flag down a security guard from the club to escort you. But remember, you don't really know who this security guard is, so be careful whom you choose. Devices can be slipped in your handbag or jacket or placed on cars to track you.

   I taught my young daughter that in a crowd she should pre-pick people to go to for help should we become separated. I taught her to go into a shop and look for a lady behind the counter. Women are much safer than men to approach. They will help you find the right people.

9. Social media is evil lurking. Sharing with the world every little thing about you and where you are pretty much allows

anyone in the world to track you. Now, that is pretty scary. Think about it: anyone has access to you anytime they want. Remove your personal life from all social media and save it for your true friends and partners. The people on the internet are not your real friends. People pretend to be people they are not in order take advantage of others mentally, emotionally, physically, sexually, financially. Don't be a victim. Be proactive and guard yourself.

10. Human trafficking is a real thing. People are kidnapped all the time for sexual and physical slavery and harvesting of human organs. Some parents will drop their children off in places, thinking the kids are safe because they have cell phones. That is not the case. All someone has to do is grab the kid, drug them so they can't function, toss their phone, and remove the kid from the premises. Poof. Gone in an instant. These people might wake up in another country with no identification, and may not even speak the same language. Girls and boys, your cell phones are tracking devices, but they don't protect you from acts of violence, rape, kidnapping, abuse, etc.

11. Your phones really are only good for phone calls, making appointments, and occasional research. Have you ever noticed something you were thinking about showing up on your phone—and you didn't even type it in the search engine? Well, I would say that is artificial intelligence using neuromarketing, picking up brain patterns, facial cues, and frequencies so it can monitor and track your every thought. How scary is that? Our phones can read our minds and send messages to us, good or bad. This is how enterprises manipulate you and the way you think and feel. If you feel you are overweight, then all these weight-loss advertisements come up, feeding you the message that you should not feel okay within yourself.

You are perfect just the way you are. Turn off your phones

and stay away from advertisements. You are being brainwashed all day, every day.

In the middle of the night, I was listening to a healing meditation app only to be interrupted with an advertisement for Lyme disease. What? Who in their right mind would insert a negative thinking pattern right into this healing meditation? I practically screamed. I couldn't stop thinking about illness when I was working so hard to clear myself from all illness. If I had fallen asleep, imagine what kind of imprint that would have had on my subconscious brain.

Get it? Our brains are being programmed. See, hear, and feel what I am talking about here. Technology is ruining our society if not monitored properly. It hits you consciously, subconsciously, and unconsciously. There may come a day when most people flee the cities and prefer to live a more "off the grid" lifestyle in order to have peace and get away from technology. You might love it today, but in the future, you may realize it really messed up your life.

• • •

## DIVORCE

There is a really good chance your parents, you, a friend, or someone in your family will go through a divorce. The odds are against us. People grow apart, learn lessons, change, redesign their lives, redirect their attention, get sidetracked, make bad choices, abuse drugs/alcohol, abuse one another, try to control each other, go back to childhood traumas that still need to be healed, become their toxic parents, can't see the other person's point of view, become religious, only care about themselves, and the list goes on.

It is better to separate from someone who does not accept you, align with you, support who you are, or help you evolve into a higher version of yourself. Parents have different parenting styles, beliefs, viewpoints, ethics, and values that sometimes don't appear until years or even decades later. If one doesn't think the other is pulling their weight or doing something the right way, manipulation and control might take place. This is why there is such a tug-of-war when people divorce.

Parents divorce because that time with each other is over; they each have issues they need to work out, and they can't do it if the other person is telling them how to think and behave. In order for them to grow and evolve, they need space. I know a lot of you want your parents to get back together, but if they reached this point, it really is for the best that they are apart.

This is also a time for you to expand yourself. You might have more freedom and opportunities to make decisions for yourself if they are focused more on the divorce and personal growth and less on you. Yes, I am sure you would like their attention, but good attention is the goal. For a while, your parents will be off balance. One parent might try to pit you against the other parent. Don't let them do this to you if you can help it. One is not necessarily better than the other; we are all trying to survive and thrive here. Give them space to clear and heal.

Most of all, give your parents a break. This is one of the most challenging times in their lives. They are trying to figure out how to do it all on their own, possibly on very little money. They are reinventing themselves and defining what is important to them. New partners may come in and distract them, but that is not the answer. They need to go within and heal, reflect, and repair in a process I call R to the 8th (infinite) power:

1. Retreat
2. Rest
3. Relax
4. Release
5. Repair
6. Reset

7. Recharge
8. Realign

I have done this cycle many times to heal and will cover more of this in the healing section of this book.

I believe that in the future fewer people will choose to marry due to the hardship divorce creates. However, for certain people, there is only one right mate for life, according to their DNA—just like in the movie *Avatar*.

## DEPRESSION

Many of us will experience depression multiple times in our lifetime. Things happen and life changes in ways we are not prepared for. When a loved one dies, someone we care about is diagnosed with a disorder, we suffer through a divorce or loss of a job, or someone betrays us, it takes time to wrap our mind around what has happened and to heal. That is when you go within yourself and reevaluate your entire existence—what is important to you, what you will and will not tolerate. I call this going into the storm.

I was in a depression storm for what felt like years in order to process, realign, and redirect myself to be reborn into a newer, better, higher version of me. I spend a lot of my time alone, reading, writing, and researching to understand human behavior and why I did the things I did as well as understand other people's motivations. People would say, "Take this drug to numb you." Nope. How are you supposed to heal if you are numb? You gotta go right in the storm to clean and clear and learn the lesson so you can come out and create.

When you are in the middle of the storm, write and release. Use two of those dollar-store journals I suggested you buy in the introduction—one for gratitude and one for release. Use the gratitude one every day to write three to five things you are grateful for, even if you write the same thing over and over. Use the other journal to release and let out your frustrations. Write down things that upset you, how you are feeling, what you are thinking.

I gave my daughter journals at a very young age and suggested she write what she was thinking and feeling. She ended up creating a journal wherein she dedicated each page to one person in her life. She would maybe write their astrological sign, what they liked to eat, how they behaved, how they thought, what they were good at. It was rather incredible. She evaluated each person's strengths and weaknesses all on her own. She also created journals for TV shows, songs she liked, feelings, ideas, etc. The possibilities are endless.

That is what journaling is for: to let it all out. You don't have to show it to anyone. But you may notice you tend to carry a pattern, and it is those patterns you learn from. There is something about taking a pen to paper rather than typing on the computer. You will see what I mean when you get the hang of it and make it a habit.

You can have all the money in the world, but if you are alone and have lost hope, you might feel you have nothing. People don't understand this. They think if you have this or that, you should never feel depressed. How people treat you and make you think and feel is the culprit here. In trying to please others, we often sacrifice ourselves, our health, and our happiness. There is no way to please everyone.

We like to think that if we are smart, perfect, and have it all together, we are lovable. But the truth is that you have to love yourself first. People may call you selfish for doing that, but remember: when you fly with an airline, the flight attendants say to put your oxygen mask on first before you assist others. The same goes for depression. You need to go within to heal and love yourself and do whatever it takes to get through the storm. And different ways of healing work for different people. Additionally, what works for you today may not work for you tomorrow, so be prepared to constantly evolve and try new things. This means life will never be boring.

## THE GRIEVING PROCESS

They say there are five to seven stages of grief. I consider grieving as processing new information that we have not had to deal with before. Some events can be so traumatic that they bring us down for a while. I would like to cover the stages here so you are knowledgeable about them.

1. Shock and denial
2. Pain and guilt
3. Anger and bargaining
4. Depression, loneliness, and reflection
5. Upward turn
6. Reconstruction
7. Acceptance and hope

You will grieve in your lifetime. Things happen out of your control. There are entire books and groups devoted to this topic. I suggest reading and seeking out support groups for guidance when going through heavy-duty healing.

## FAILURE

Every time I hear about a useful tactic or product, I try to incorporate it into my life.

Sara Blakely, the girl who invented Spanx, was speaking at a seminar. Her story is inspiring. She talked about how her dad insisted she had to fail at something every day—because if she didn't fail at something, it meant she didn't even try. So when she came home from school, her dad would ask her, "What did you fail at today?" And Sara would tell him something she had tried and failed to do. When she didn't have an incident to share with him, he would pry something out of her.

He was teaching her that failure was a given when lessons were learned. You can only learn if you fail, and you will eventually learn to succeed by figuring out what works and doesn't. I loved this analogy and incorporated it into my life with my daughter. I didn't have a dad to give me this kind of guidance at that stage in my life, so I took this dad's guidance and am giving it to you now. Get out there and fail your butt off. Fake it till you make it.

## BEATING YOURSELF UP

A lot of us spend a good portion of our lives beating ourselves up. I know women who are still doing it in their fifties. And you know what I learned about this? You are your number one cheerleader. If you continue to beat yourself up, you will be the one preventing you from accomplishing your goals and dreams.

In order to combat this issue, I went into complete self-love and self-care for months at a time. By doing this, you are giving your soul exactly what it needs. Only you know what you need. I nurtured myself with the right foods, exercise, nature, and safe environment, and I kept to myself. I distanced myself from friends, family, and neighbors. This way, my own energy was allowed to blossom and flourish without anyone interfering and telling me I was doing things wrong or pushing their ways on me. I started whispering or yelling to myself, "I love you, Noelle. I am proud of you, Noelle." I did this because I heard, felt, and realized that the only person I could count on and trust is myself.

So whenever you need a pick-me-up, imagine something amazing you want in your life—and then become it and create it for yourself. I did this many times just by watering my garden. I think my plants loved me back as I watched them blossom and become radiant.

## SUICIDE

There may come a point in your life when you think and feel like you are better off removing yourself from this planet. We are often flooded with strong emotions and frustration from overwhelming situations; sometimes we just want to make it all stop.

My best friend from high school committed suicide. She was facing a divorce from a man who cheated on her and embezzled money from their business. She lost everything. She sold all her designer clothes, handbags, and was getting ready to sell her beautiful home on a hill with its breathtaking views when she took her life. I later discovered she was doing drugs and drinking. She had been on a downward slope. She had attempted suicide in the past by stabbing herself in the heart. I believe she did this due to a broken heart.

My friend was one of the most giving women I ever knew. She was loving, kind, and sensitive. As teens we hung out because we both had hard family lives, and she still carried the tragedy of hers with her. She was always trying to please her mom, who could never be pleased; her mom was unpredictable and abused her mentally and emotionally. My friend always had to look perfect and be perfect, which is an impossible goal for anyone.

I truly believe suicide comes into play when your soul wants to leave the body—due to what others are doing to us, what has been done to us, what we have done to ourselves, and what we have allowed to happen to us. You see no way out; you lose hope. You want to make it all stop now.

Your body is telling you it is way off course; the soul is not in alignment with its true purpose. What your soul needs is realignment and healing. A new mission and purpose is rising. You are usually in the midst of a huge transformational storm. You are either going to survive and then thrive, or you are going to give up.

If you are contemplating suicide, this is the time to decide what drastic changes you are going to make to your life to get in alignment with who you are and what you are here to do. I believe you feel overwhelmed because you are in an environment, situation, or predicament you are supposed to outmaneuver and redirect your attention and purpose to. It's very uncomfortable when confronted, which pushes you to a breaking point. But the magic lies in overcoming it.

Also keep in mind that people have hormonal and chemical imbalances from 5G radiation, improper nutrition, lack of sleep, lack of vitamins and supplements, lack of sunshine, body toxins, energy hijackers, etc. This can really have an impact on the way we are thinking and feeling. Get your butt outside and power up your energy with the healing effects of Mother Nature.

• • •

## OTHER BEHAVIORS TO IDENTIFY

### Passive-Aggressive

Passive-aggressive behavior is a pattern of indirectly expressing negative feelings instead of being open with them. There's a disconnect between a person's behavior and what they say, which can make it hard to identify. I find people who are very sarcastic tend to be passive-aggressive. They use this technique to openly jab at people through a joking approach. In actuality, they are trying to hurt you out of resentment. You can do more research on this subject if you feel someone around you is exhibiting it.

### Bipolar

Bipolar disorder, also known as manic depression, is a mental health condition that causes extreme mood swings. People with bipolar disorder experience episodes of severe depression and episodes of mania. Mania often manifests in overwhelming joy, happiness, excitement, energy surges, a feeling of reduced need for sleep, and subdued inhibitions. No two people have the exact same tendencies. There is no known cause of bipolar disorder, but a mixture of chemistry, genetics, altered states of the brain (from drugs and alcohol, for example, which manipulate emotions to extremes), and environment are said to play a part.

## Borderline Personality Disorder

Borderline personality disorder is considered a mental health disorder that impacts the way you think and feel about yourself and others. You have an intense fear of abandonment or instability, and you may have difficulty tolerating being alone. Impulsiveness, anger, and mood swings may push others away even as you desire lasting and loving relationships.

## Post-traumatic Stress Disorder

Also known as PTSD. Post-traumatic stress disorder is a mental health condition that's triggered by a terrifying event, either experiencing it or witnessing it. PTSD may last for months or years, with triggers that can bring back memories of the trauma accompanied by intense mental, physical, and emotional responses. Symptoms may include heightened reactions, depression, moodiness, nightmares, memories of the trauma, and avoidance of situations that bring back memories of the trauma. A lot of soldiers suffer from this after experiencing violence. Children might suffer this after witnessing something devastating happening to a parent or family member. Others suffer from this after a rape, a loss of something valuable to them, graphic violence, or other unimaginable circumstances. The pandemic has caused a lot of PTSD in the community and world.

## Attention-Deficit Disorder and Attention-Deficient Hyperactivity Disorder

Attention-deficit disorder is diagnosed if a kid under age sixteen has six or more of the following symptoms for six months in a row:

1. Impulsiveness
2. Disorganization and problems prioritizing
3. Poor time-management skills
4. Problems focusing on a task

5. Trouble multitasking
6. Excessive activity or restlessness
7. Poor planning
8. Low frustration tolerance
9. Frequent mood swings
10. Problems following through and completing tasks
11. Hot temper
12. Trouble coping with stress

ADHD is diagnosed only when symptoms are severe enough to cause ongoing problems in more than one area of your life. These continuous symptoms can be traced back to early childhood years. Now do you see why it is really important to be able to analyze our home living situations and how we are parenting and are parented?

## Narcissistic Personality Disorder

Narcissists are selfish people with a sense of entitlement. They may lack empathy and desire admiration. Musicians and other famous and successful people often carry this trait. They are very charming and likable at first. They will come on strong, use compliments, draw you in and hook you, make you feel good like a drug does, and then remove their love and affection from you. It is intoxicating and toxic at the same time, as well as confusing and compromising to your soul.

Narcissists prey upon empaths because empaths are very giving. They will suck the life force out of you if you let them—by making you feel bad, using manipulative behavior, acting as if they are always right and that they know better and you are wrong or incompetent. If you fall in love with a narcissistic person, you will go through many emotions once the relationship is over. Be prepared to deal with the roller coaster ride for a little while before you gain your bearings once again.

### Parent Alienation

Parent alienation is when one parent psychologically manipulates their child to look negatively on the other parent. Basically, it's a form of brainwashing for the conscious and unconscious mind. I do find that kids who suffer from this abuse have depression and thoughts of suicide due to the confusion it causes. Please don't do this to your children or allow your parents to do this with you. It is very damaging to the soul because kids shares genes with both parents, bringing on massive amounts of guilt, fear, and stress.

• • •

## ELECTROMAGNETIC FIELDS

An electromagnetic field is a classical field produced by accelerating electric charges. These are also known as EMF. Did you know all your electronic devices are giving off EMF? Your Wi-Fi, your phone, your TV, your laptop—it is everywhere, and it's on full blast. In listening to international podcasts, I discovered many other countries are boycotting 5G networks. Not here in the US. Here they pop up like flowers. Scientists used to say there is no evidence to conclude that exposure to low-level electromagnetic fields is harmful to human health, but we are finding that is not true. I have heard of families living beside powerlines whose children ended up with brain tumors and health problems many years after the lines were built. We will talk more about this later in the book.

## MOTHER EARTH'S HEALING FIELDS

Recently the city I have lived in for over thirty years undertook what they called "neighborhood beautification." They converted our sidewalk corners to accommodate the upcoming remote-control Amazon delivery wagon robot, claiming the changes were for wheelchair access. But when you see men testing these wagon robots throughout the neighborhood and noting ways to accommodate them, you tend to notice.

The city also came in and removed fifteen fifty-year-old trees, jacking up the ecosystem. You see, under the ground, trees talk to each other through a network somewhat like the internet. It was all disrupted, causing major chaos. My house was invaded by rats looking for a new home.

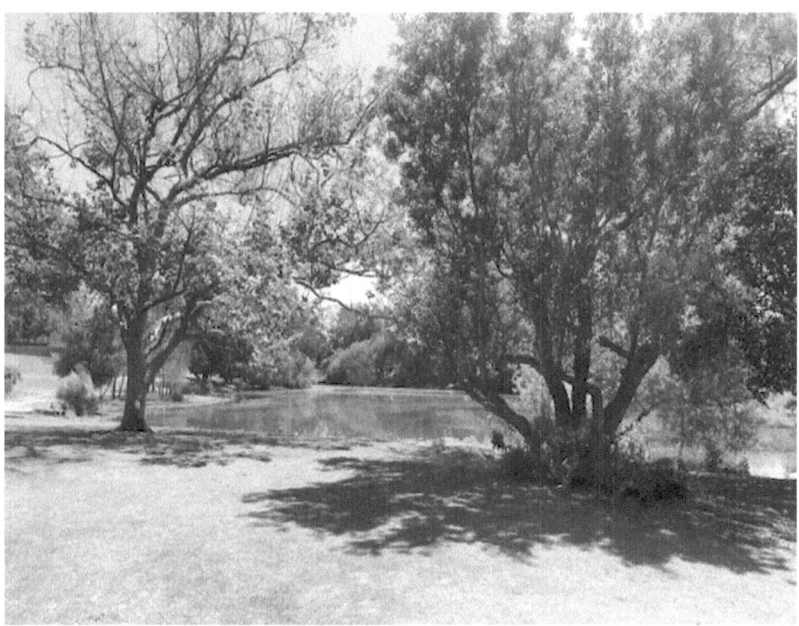

Those trees that had created a healing field that protected our families and our homes from 5G electromagnetic energy were simply gone.

Our entire neighborhood felt an instant shift from the good, vibrant energy of Mother Earth to darkness and doom. We were disturbed by the dramatic actions. None of us had been notified. My daughter and I cried for the trees and the loss of their healing force field. Our beautiful, tree-lined streets now looked like bowling alley lanes with light poles.

I want you to pay attention to this. You can't put back Mother

Nature. Sure, the city is going to plant new trees. But they will never be as big and beautiful and healthy as the previous ones. These new trees will have been doused with 5G radiation and toxins that didn't exist on this planet fifty years ago when there were fewer cars, fewer people, and less pollution. Those trees had withstood the test of time, had acquired wisdom and knowledge by occupying the space for so long and witnessing us and protecting us. Those trees communicated with one another under the ground and with each of us as well as preserving Mother Nature, wildlife, and high vibrational healing frequencies.

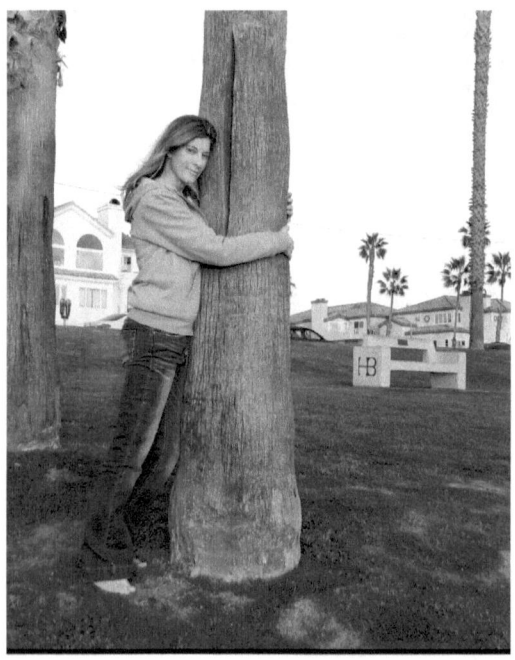

When people want to come in and tear things down to put in new developments and structures or to accommodate technology, pay attention to the underlying factors. Is this accommodating artificial intelligence or human survival? Or both? Many people care more for money than the well-being of society. Mother Nature is the key to our living healthy lives for a very long time. Her needs have been ignored for thousands of years in the name of evolution. We can only beat her up for so long before she fights back or gives up on us.

Respect Mother Nature, and she will love you back unconditionally, grant you healing forces, and fill you with wisdom. Stepping out into her will heal you from 5G, radiation, technology overload, and energy blockages and will help you enhance your superpowers. Don't let anyone take Mother Nature away.

## LEVELING UP

When you are leveling up, you are in transition, opening yourself to an epiphany that may hit like lightning. This will allow you to see things from several perspectives, not just your own. Leveling up means you are pushing through your boundaries as well as others' ideas on limitations. You are creating instead of endlessly following. You are moving to the next level in the game of life.

## LEARN TO IDENTIFY TOXICITY

I want you to empower yourself with the ability to identify toxic behaviors, toxic environments, and unhealthy situations from a young age. When you are young, you typically cannot identify these behaviors and patterns because no one has sat down and explained them to you; you also might not have encountered them yet. You might experience a lot of unhealthy situations that will affect you for the rest of your life if you don't take the time to listen, read, comprehend, and understand what can lead to them.

By journaling, you can document your feelings and emotions and get in touch with your senses to identify what is actually taking place. It is usually not until you have had the negative experience or gone through a traumatic event that you realize and learn the lesson and clear the karma.

It seems to me society has thrown out morals, values, and ethics, and we need to establish some guidelines and boundaries for ourselves and others. Be aware that you are going to experience strange and unhealthy behaviors from those around you—those who live with you, work with you, and learn with you. These unhealthy programs have been running through humanity over many lifetimes. We also need to take into account the effect of artificial intelligence on the human soul. AI is being used to program us and redirect the way we think and behave. The goal here is to identify it sooner, cut it off, and change it. You are only responsible for the way you handle yourself. Do the best you can in any given situation, forgive yourself for the choices you make, accept others, and move forward the best way you can.

## SCHOOL COUNSELORS, MENTORS, TEACHERS, THERAPISTS

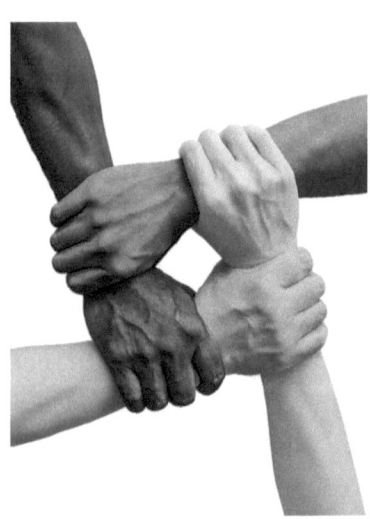

You should now realize the importance of obtaining a positive mental support system. Every single kid should have a good counselor/therapist/mentor they can talk to, if only to discuss their hopes and dreams. Now is the time to seek a professional to start guiding you on the healthiest journey you can create for yourself. You can and will create amazing things. Clear your path to access your superpowers.

## JOURNAL: Chapter 3

1. Write down types of abuse you have noticed. Break it down by . . .
    A. Elementary school
    B. Junior high
    C. High school
    D. Home life

    Call out anybody and everybody who has done anything to bother you.

2. Write down anything you want to release regarding the negative behaviors you have noticed taking place.

3. Write down ways you wish you'd handled the situation better. What could you do now that you know? Come up with solutions for the future should the situation arise again.

Gratitude Journal: From this point on you, will be writing every day in your gratitude journal. Take out your gratitude journal and write three to five things that you are grateful for. When you do this, you attract good things and realize you have a lot to be thankful for. Your vibration will rise when gratitude attitude is projected, felt, and aligned. Journaling gratitude is one of the most important things you can do. It has accelerated healing effects!

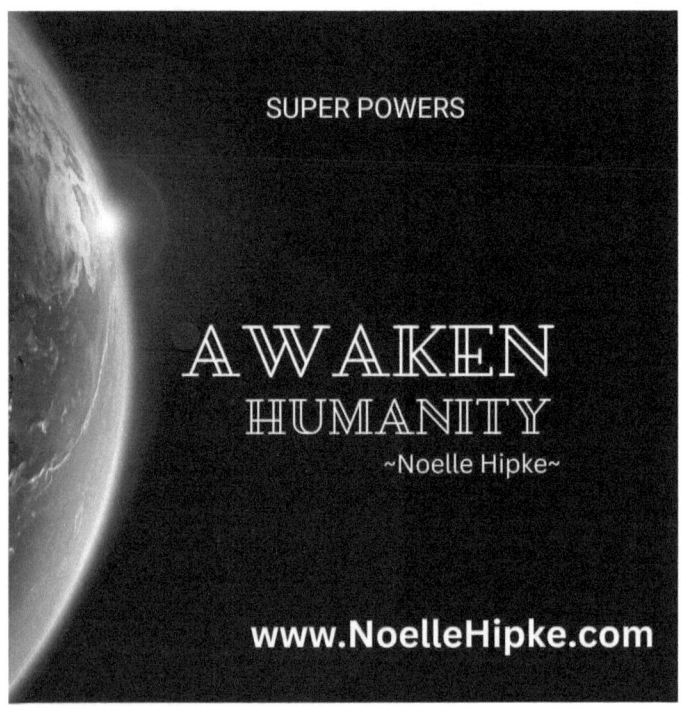

## CHAPTER FOUR

# THE ENERGETIC BODY

## WHAT IS ENERGY IN THE BODY?

The human body contains enormous quantities of energy. Electrical energy sends signals and nerve impulses back and forth to our brains, and thermal energy helps us to maintain body temperature, while mechanical energy helps us to move. The human body runs off chemical energy. This energy comes from the foods we eat. Bodies digest the food by mixing it with acids and enzyme fluids in the stomach. Eating the right foods for our body type will aid digestion and produce energy. The average adult has as much energy stored in fat as a one-ton battery produces.

A human's health is determined by our electric health, so you are going to really want to pay attention to how your body is storing, using, and manipulating energy. As we move away from a materialistic world to the energetic world of the new earth, you will see a transformational change of focus for humanity.

### Auras

Auras are seen as bubbles that reflect the vibrational energy of every living being—including plants, animals, and even Mother Nature herself—and come in different strengths and colors. When in alignment I can see the colors and energies of people's auras, allowing me to gather information about how the person is feeling or the shape of their health. Auras extend out three to five feet beyond the body to reveal frequency, spirit, and personality and consist of seven layers. The first layer syncs to security and health of the physical body, relating to manifestation. The second layer pertains to emotions and boundaries. The third layer correlates to basic beliefs, personal power, intellect, self-understanding, as well as understanding of others. The fourth layer connects to relationships and love in general, such as self-love, love of your body, your loved ones. The fifth layer relates to your uniqueness and inner identity as they relate to communication. The sixth layer highlights group consciousness, nonlinear intellect, belief systems, clairvoyance, and forms of higher unconditional love. The seventh layer is your spiritual guide, a.k.a. higher self. Each layer has its own energetic frequency.

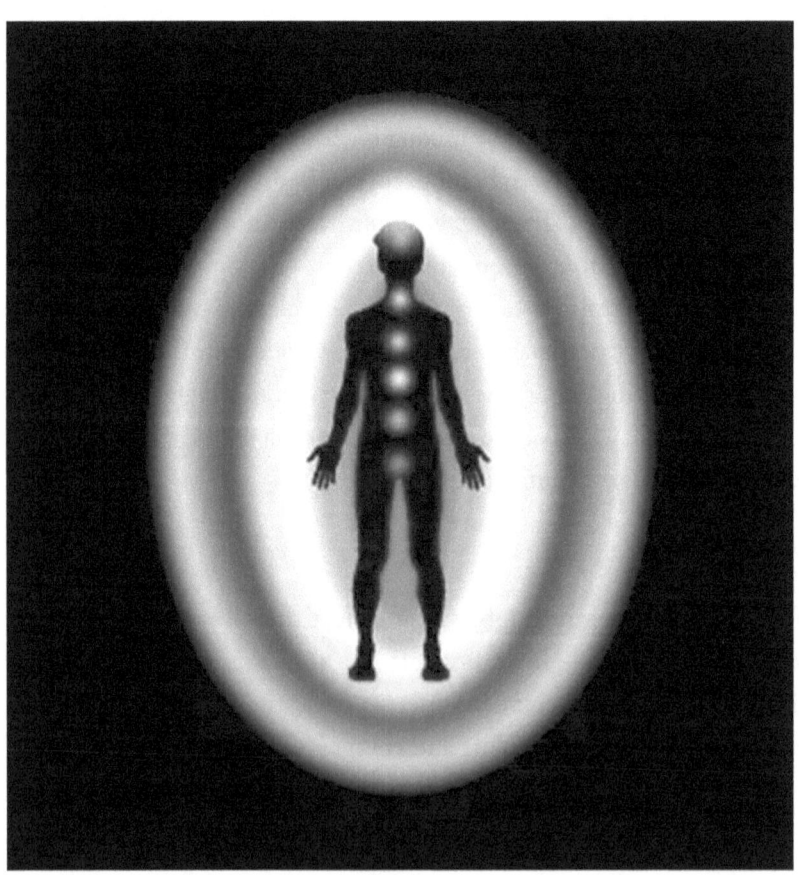

When you personally move into higher frequencies from 3D to 5D, you can see and sense other people's auras based on the frequency of energy they are emitting and broadcasting. Your aura is connected to your chakra system, which is connected to your rainbow light body. Your rainbow light body is what your soul transforms into when it is reaching higher states of consciousness, which in turn moves you into ascension. Humans who heal and protect their energetic auras reach these higher levels of consciousness to achieve the ultimate goal of ascension. Ascension is energy moving into higher frequencies and maintaining it.

## Force Field

Our force field is an invisible boundary of exerted strength consisting of sensory field, charisma, or energetic influence toward others. A force field monitors movement toward an area or object.

## Biofield

The biofield has recently gained a lot of traction when it comes to determining the state of one's well-being, mind, and life force and may very well be the new frontier in healthcare. The biofield is the energy field that surrounds and extends out from the body around eight feet and can be felt with the hands through pressure and temperature changes. The biofield is composed of measurable electromagnetic energy, chi, and subtle energy.

Special devices like the Bio-Well can measure a person's biofield by assessing the energetic state of a being. The device can tell if someone has been damaged. Our biofield can become impaired due to a multiplication of negative energy, negative thinking, negative arrows and energy from others, negative feelings and emotions, bad environment, poor nutrition and health complications, misalignment of the chakras, and disconnection of the meridians, among other things.

The human body is complex and well beyond what we previously imagined. It releases acoustic energy, low-level light, and heat. Humans can convert energy and have electromagnetic properties that can't be defined by chemistry or physics. Technology and evolution now bring to the forefront what others have dismissed as hocus pocus. People always want to measure or prove anything that is invisible to the human eye doesn't exist, even if they are not paying attention or seeking to see the unseen. However, we can actually see this field. Ever watch someone who is really angry? You can read, see, and feel their energy in their eyes, on their face, in their body language. They will suck the life force out of you if you let them.

Understanding the biofield effects a positive change in people's health and well-being by creating space to discover a deeper level of coherency and communication between cells, tissues, organs, and physical systems.

What I have learned about the biofield:

- It is the human energy field/aura.
- It is an electric current with a magnetic field.
- It is the body's electrical system.
- It extends eight feet around the body.
- It senses the atmosphere around our body.
- It holds coding and genetic patterns.
- It contains knowledge you have gained over lifetimes.
- It protects our well-being.
- Fear creates a certain pulse and causes twice the amount of energy in the system.
- Fear—misuse of energy—causes humans to stop perceiving things clearly.
- Depression has a low vibration.

## Chakras

I have been studying the chakras for decades, and this concept is finally being backed up by science thanks to new technologies. What I want you to take away from this is that there are just some things you know and believe that others will not. This book is meant to show you how to enter into higher levels and frequencies to tap into this unlimited, invisible information of ascension. Others may not be able to access the superpower levels you have achieved.

Chakras are used in ancient meditation practices in the tradition of Hinduism. Here we go again, delving into other cultures, traditions, and religions. Many people tend to shut out teachings if they don't believe or trust the parent religion or culture, which prevents them from putting the pieces together and realizing that we are all one in unconditional love.

Chakras are vortices of spinning energy located in our etheric body on the midline of the spine. Energy is known as chi, prana, life force, or vital energy. There are seven primary chakras connected to various functions that keep our spiritual, mental, physical, and emotional health in balance. When all of your chakras are open and you are clear and balanced, the magic of the universe floods you with a state of well-being.

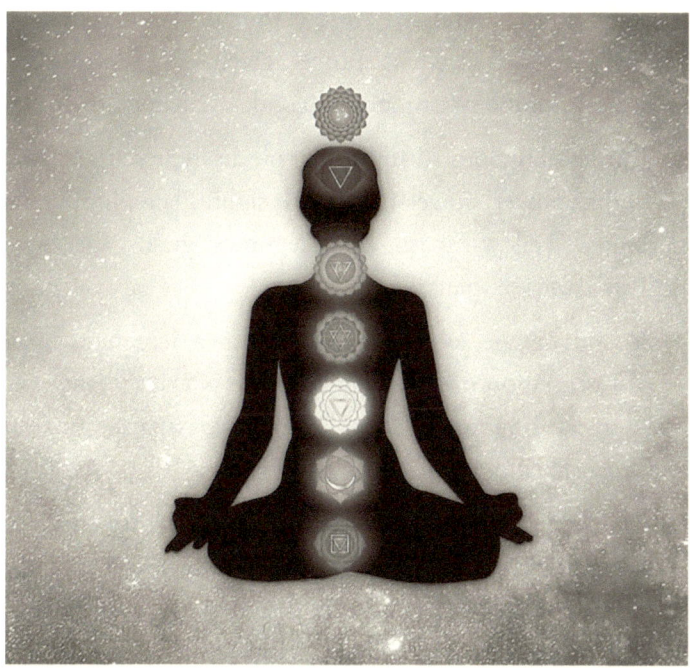

Each chakra has a special purpose, color, element, symbol, sense, crystal, food, action, planet, and sound:

- Seventh: purple, located at the crown of the head; represents conscious enlightenment; the related sense is will. Moon Planet.
- Sixth: indigo, located at the third eye; represents awareness, intuition, perception, transcendence; the related sense is clairvoyant and extrasensory perception. Sun Planet. Foods: blackberries, plums, grapes. Organs: pituitary gland, forehead, temples.
- Fifth: blue, located at the throat; represents communication, self-expression, inner truth; the related sense is sound. Planet Mercury. Foods: blueberries, plumbs, soups, sea vegetables. Organs: thyroid, throat, mouth.
- Fourth: green, located at the heart; represents balance, love, body, spirit; the related sense is touch. Planet Venus. Foods; limes, kiwis, honeydew, sprouts, green leafy veggies. Organs: heart, immune system, lungs, blood, circulatory, thymus.
- Third: yellow, located at the solar plexus; represents self-esteem, vitality, power; the related sense is sight. Planet Jupiter. Foods: lemons, yellow squash, corn, legumes, grains. Organs: eyes, liver, stomach, pancreas.
- Second: orange, located at the pelvic area; represents creativity, passion, emotions; the related sense is taste. Planet Saturn. Foods: cantaloupes, carrots, oranges, papaya, nuts, seeds. Organs: bladder, gonads, sexual organs.
- First: red, located at the root of spine; represents security, survival, instinct, grounding; the related sense is smell. Planet Mars. Foods: beets, cherries, red cabbage, root vegetables. Organs: teeth, bones, adrenal glands, kidneys.

When your chakras are in complete alignment, your superpowers are in full force. Intuition and clairvoyant abilities are heightened and so are all your senses, creating a sense of oneness.

## Out-of-Body Chakras

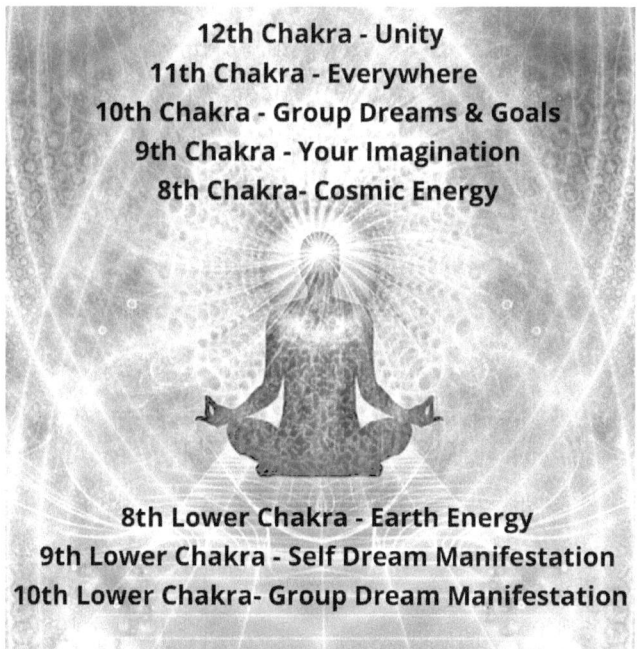

Okay, I am going to take you up another level here. Besides the basic chakras you may have encountered, there are also out-of-body chakras I want to make you aware of.

Chakras above the body:

- Twelfth: represents unity as one
- Eleventh: located everywhere; represents your relationship with all that is
- Tenth: located four feet above your head; represents dreams and goals for a group

- Ninth: located three feet above your head; represents what you can imagine for yourself
- Eighth: located one foot above your head; represents the multidimensional eternal self, which transforms cosmic energy

Chakras below the body:

- Eighth: located one foot below; represents earth energy
- Ninth: located three feet below; represents manifesting self-dreams
- Tenth: located four feet below; represents manifesting group dreams

I went into these extended chakras while writing this book. Being in this realm helped me tap into the knowledge I needed to share with you. I had to align, clear, clean, connect, transcend, ascend, listen, and release all at the same time in order to access my superpowers and bring you this content.

You all can do this if you work with the writings I have shared with you in this book. Many other people have accessed these same realms to gather knowledge and wisdom and bring about innovative concepts and technology.

• • •

## WE ARE ENERGY

Our bodies are magnificent energy generators. I have literally blown out light bulbs and speakers in my home when lifting my energetic vibration to high levels. It's like I am a lightning bolt when I activate my superpowers and am in alignment with my force field, biofield, and chakras.

I consider these to be our six inherent powers:

1. Purity is power
2. Positivity is power
3. Plants are power
4. People are power
5. Pleasure is power
6. Peace is power

Men have told me that I have electrocuted them when we kiss. You know why? Because I am careful about who I share my energy with. I only share with the right people.

I have learned that when you are a lightworker, people are drawn to you like moths to a flame. Before I learned to safeguard my energy, I could attract men but often not the kind of men I wanted to entertain. Rather, these were usually men who needed to work on themselves, heal, and clear their energy; they only wanted to be serviced, have sex, be worshipped, or be taken care of.

I could immediately see when they were not centered. As my superpowers enhanced, I became better at reading people, their frequency, and their energy. I could read it in their online profiles photos, and I could see it in their eyes, their skin, their face, and their body. I grew so good at this that my friends often sent me photos of men they were going to meet to see if I could get a reading.

If I saw men surrounded by photos of their cars, boats, and materialistic things, I knew they were only looking for a pretty girl. They were promoting their lifestyle and success—which they most likely had—but didn't know how to treat people or had not worked on themselves, which was why they were alone.

Of course, many wealthy men are alone. And many wealthy women are alone. And I believe many more people will choose to live this way. Why? For some people, it is easier to be alone in your own beautiful biofield of energy. You can heal yourself, stay centered, and no one will come in to zap you of your energy and manipulate you.

There is great power in being alone. I have spent the last three years alone, working on myself.

When this pandemic hit, it was a wake-up call to heal ourselves on very deep levels, break patterns, and bring awareness to the inner aspects that needed attention. When you are alone, you can fart, belch, release, scream, laugh at yourself, talk to yourself, watch whatever you want on TV, and sleep in the middle of the bed. However, we are not all meant to be alone forever. We are meant to share our amazing energy with each other. But there may come a time when you just have to shut out the world so you can align with your higher self.

This is one of the healthiest things you can do. It prevents you from looking to others for validation, acceptance, and appreciation. You go within to create self-love and find self-sufficient ways to fill your own cup with healing energy. This is how you truly heal yourself: spending time alone to listen, understand, comprehend, and draw awareness to your inner self. When you heal the inner self, you heal your soul. Sure, your soul is going to have ups and downs, and this is a constant process. But the goal is to be aware of what is taking place so you can make little tweaks to get aligned.

## PEMF THERAPY MATS

As I have mentioned, I'm going to repeat several topics throughout, and here I'm going to address PEMF mats again. Pulsed electromagnetic mat field therapy is holistic therapy used by healers, doctors, chiropractors, cardiologists, athletic trainers, and physical therapists, and can be found in hospitals, ambulances, and other healing centers around the world.

PEMF brings electricity into the body to align the body, mind, and soul on a cellular level. Since we are made of energy, this process is like recharging and recalibrating our internal battery. I think of it as sound-frequency healing, only we can't really hear it. Our pets can hear it, and I hear it on occasion when I am using the mat, but for the most part it is silent to the human ear (just like 5G and other radiation devices).

I truly believe sound frequency is going to be our ultimate source of healing the body now and in the future. I will cover more on this later in the book.

Judging by my experience and research, PEMF devices help us realign our DNA and organs, purify our blood, and clear our biofield by sending magnetic energy into the body to enhance the body's natural magnetic field. These mats are the newest frontier in self-healing therapy. We are all going to need PEMF due to the invisible energies surrounding us on a daily basis. When you are sitting in a classroom of thirty people, you have at least thirty phones on in the room, and the 5G and radiation from all those phones is going right through your body, mind, soul, and cells. Add in computers, tablets, and teaching platforms, and the amount of radiation is off the charts.

Nobody wants to talk about how all these 5G and radiation devices may be damaging us. Instead they want to promote more devices, newer phones, wireless this, and wireless that. Sleeping on a PEMF mat at night can help clear the EMF harm that has been done to your body during the day. Damaged or injured areas of the human body can be sensed and now seen in biofield readings thanks to technology that can detect deficiencies.

I believe that at some point you are going to need to consider obtaining PEMF therapy to combat the electrical toxicity we face. Electrical toxicity is so far an invisible grid surrounding us. Just imagine what it would look like if you could see it.

## HOBBIES ENERGIZE

You might find yourself taking up a new hobby or going back to something you used to do as a kid. In my fifties, my ten-year-old daughter saw a girl twirling a baton on YouTube and asked if she could get one. I used to twirl a baton when I was her age, so I ordered one for me and one for her. It was like riding a bike. When I picked up the baton and twirled it, I felt like a ten-year-old kid again. It was pure magic. Twirling my baton has been one of the most freeing activities for me ever since. My friend was at my house when it arrived and asked me if I had led a parade, which of course I had not. Back in my day, my hobby consisted of me roller skating around and twirling my baton. But I will take the compliment, thank you very much.

Finding a hobby that "lights you up" will help you regain energetic alignment. The cells in my body tingled when I twirled, danced, sang, and put myself into the highest form of vibration I could create for myself. Little girls waved, people watched, and I released, recharged, and regenerated my body, mind, and soul.

So the ultimate goal for you is to find something like this that makes your soul sing. It could be playing an instrument, dirt biking, exercising, gardening, or simply walking. Find an activity that makes you tingle. That means you are on the right track.

This is what I want you to realize. Our energetic bodies are so powerful when we treat them right and give them exactly what they need. Everyone needs something different because we are all unique. Your body will direct you; all you have to do is listen. That is why meditation is so important, and so is peace and quiet. You need to slow down the body and mind in order to receive the information and messages your body and higher self are trying to communicate to you. You can't muck it up with drugs, alcohol, and crappy foods. You have to make sure you are detoxed, eating clean, flushing out the toxins, drinking living water, and aligning yourself to become one with nature and nurture your inner being. When you do all these things, you radiate and set your superpowers in motion.

Let's talk again about the biofield. People will poke holes in your biofield; that's what bullies and jealous, uneducated, judgmental, or toxic people in general do. Themselves unaligned, they want to steal your radiant energy. Maybe they don't know how to align, don't care to do it, or don't believe in it. You can't let the way others think and behave determine how you are going to feel and respond.

I suggest getting away from people and situations that don't attract the right energy. You might not have a choice when it comes to being stuck in classroom and work situations, but you can be selective in how you spend your free time and who with. I have been in situations where the energy is so toxic that it literally made me sick on multiple levels. A lot of you may not have been paying attention, so I am here to bring this to the forefront for you: when you and those around you are aware and self-aware and someone gets out of line and misbehaves, you can all identify the toxic behavior and energy right off the bat.

Say you and your friends are all in alignment and accept each other for who you are. You appreciate each other's differences and know you each bring your own superpowers to the table. Then some kid comes out of nowhere and starts instigating problems and challenging you. You will immediately feel a change in the energy and the biofield around you.

My daughter came home really upset one day after getting attacked from behind by an older boy on the playground. She was very distraught about the encounter. I told her, "He was drawn to you and your beautiful energy. He wanted to take some of your good life force." I truly believe men who attack women are not just looking for sex. They want to enter a woman's sacred space, which is basically a gateway to her pure, angelic, energetic life force field. Ladies, this is why I state it is very important to be selective with whom you let into your internal biofield.

Our biofield sends us signals about dangers, feelings, emotions, insights, awareness, clarity, perceptions, the higher self, and transcendence when it is in alignment. That is why animals can sense a natural disaster approaching. They aren't tuning out the body's messages with electronic devices, drugs, drinking, and filling the body with toxicity. They are completely clean, clear, and aware, and their senses are on full alert. And this is the state of mind you need in order to access your superpowers and maintain a powerful force field.

Thanks to science and technology, biofield-reading devices can capture a person's energy. These powerful tools prove we are made up of energy. We may very well count on these devices in the future to detect the difference between an actual human being and an artificially intelligent human clone.

## MY SUPERPOWERS

There are things I just know in my bones. I could spend all day trying to convince someone, but that would be a waste of my good energy. I simply shrug and chuckle. They may never know nor understand the things I know, and I am okay with that. They have their own journey. You can benefit from all my years of experience or choose to ignore me. Take what resonates with you from this book and leave the rest. If I give you just one aha moment, that is what I came here to accomplish. Life is a puzzle, and we're meant to put all the pieces together—or connect the dots, as I've said.

I have been connecting the dots for five decades and notice things the average person does not. When I did the research and discovered that other humans with similar personality traits to mine make up 2 to 3 percent of the population, I was really bothered by this. People who vibrate on higher levels are often few and far between. However, I realized I vibrate at this level in order to get people to see and understand things they didn't see or comprehend before. Holistic health is the answer to human survival. As you detox, you become clean and clear and more aware. Your sensitivity to your surroundings will increase, and you will notice and feel the vibrations of the people around you as well as the environment.

My senses enhanced and amplified. My sense of smell, which is one of my dominant DNA traits, became animalistic. I was able to pick up unusual fragrances and notice things I never did before, just from a scent. I got messages from the smell of something. I could smell cancer: it smells metallic. I noticed this when I hugged someone. I could see it, feel it, and smell it in their energy field. This all showed that my force field, biofield, and superpowers were in full alignment.

All of your superpower senses will be amplified—vision, taste, hearing, touch, and smell. In turn, this will activate senses you didn't even know existed. I call this the super shift.

Here are a few of the senses you may activate when you are in alignment:

1. Clairsentience ("clear feeling"): the ability to perceive emotional or psychic energy that is imperceptible to the five standard senses
2. Claircognizance ("clear knowing"): the ability for a person to acquire knowledge without knowing how or why they know it
3. Clairvoyance ("clear seeing"): perceiving things or events in the future or beyond normal sensory contact
4. Clairalience ("clear smelling"): strong sense of smell, able to smell odors that don't have any physical source
5. Clairaudience ("clear hearing"): hearing words, music, or sounds in one's own mind that have no physical source
6. Clairgustance ("clear tasting"): heightened sense of taste, expanded taste buds
7. Telepathy ("flash perception"): communication of thoughts or ideas directly from one mind to another without speech or signs
8. Transcendence ("rising above"): existence or experience beyond the normal or physical level

Some people's DNA may allow them to access this data more easily than others, but I truly believe we all have the ability to super shift when we make the conscious decision to do so. And that is what I am here to share with you. This isn't just for healers or psychics. I am teaching you the direct way to connect and align with your higher self and how you can enhance your superpowers to go into a super-shift mindset.

What do you think you could create in the world if you had these capabilities? Don't you want to try it for yourself? Don't you wonder what it feels like to have Spidey senses? You can do this. You can create this. You can feel this. This is the future of amazing health, amazing connection, and amazing awareness. This is your wake-up call.

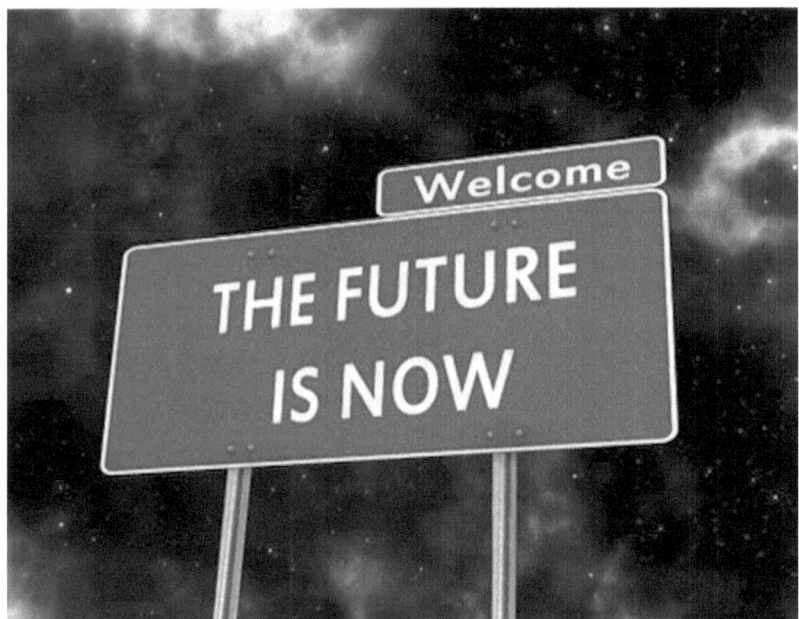

It is not taboo or lies. It is ascension, the act of rising to an important position or to a higher level. That higher level is a higher vibration on the planet.

This is the direction we are all supposed to go. You have to make the choice to step into your superpowers and super shift. We are creating a higher frequency of awareness, health, happiness, peace, joy, ease, acceptance, love, purity, patience, understanding, compassion, forgiveness, and kindness. We are all becoming one with each other, the planet, and the universe. We are like a bright star in the sky. We will be luminary.

## GROUNDING

Grounding, also known as earthing, is the act of connecting your body directly to the earth. We do this by walking barefoot on grass, sand, dirt. (All of your organs are connected to the soles of your feet—think of them as the *souls* of your feet.) The earth is hit multiple times a day with lightning, creating an energy source for all of us to tap into. You can also ground by lying on the ground and going into bodies of natural water.

When you ground and connect your body, mind, and soul to the earth, your body contacts the planet's natural electric charge. This in turn stabilizes your physiology at the deepest levels, reduces inflammation, pain, and stress, improves blood flow, energy, and sleep, and generates greater well-being. In other words, when you take the time every day to earth your energetic body system to the electrical power within the ground and realign, you activate your ability to heal.

Human bodies need nature, trees, earth, streams, rocks, flowers, and plants to live as one with optimum health. Sure, you can simply go out in nature, but to amplify the experience, you need to see it, feel it, touch it. That is why people hug trees. The high healing vibration a tree carries is supernatural.

## SMART CITIES: NOT WHAT YOU THINK

Some cities are currently being built into "smart cities," leading to the teardown of our healing fields of trees and overall removal of Mother Nature. These smart cities will impact us with 5G radiation, radiation from electronics, microwaves, vehicles, and the list goes on.

This may very well prevent us from tapping into our superpowers to activate our super shift and force fields. It could prevent us from growing our own food supply to ensure we can live healthy; there is a chance outside forces will want to control our water supply in order to control us. You might embrace this change and think it is great, but our freedom is being ripped from underneath us—for the so-called betterment of mankind. I ask you: are these cities being built for human beings or to accommodate artificially intelligent human clones?

Smart cities will make you a slave to a system. You are going to be forced to live a certain way, which may steal or diminish your superpowers and life force if not appropriately moderated. This great future is being promoted through the digital matrix of the internet. You are being manipulated. Outside forces will control the food you eat, the amount of money you have, and the healthcare you receive.

When we move from gas-powered vehicles to electric-only vehicles, you may have all your freedoms and rights taken away if you are not careful and walk right into it willingly. Think about it. What would happen if suddenly we didn't have the electricity to charge our vehicles? We have been threatened with rolling blackouts when people use too much energy running their air-conditioning during the hot summer months, which would likewise prevent access to electricity to charge our vehicles, basically leaving us stranded or imprisoned in our homes or workspaces.

And if you think that electric vehicle isn't sending off a negative frequency and affecting your body's force field and biofield, think again. Most newer vehicles already run on computers and could very well contain an implanted device that when switched off from an external source stops the vehicle from working altogether, making it easy to debilitate society and create an uproar and outbreak of madness, fear, violence, and panic. Imagine that. Outside forces are giving us all the signs of this type of manipulation and control in bits and pieces. We need to pay attention, listen up, make better choices, change the way we do things, and alter our own course.

The younger generations have no idea what life was like when you had the freedom to choose for yourself. I want all younger generations to be very aware of this. Older forces right now are deciding what to do with your life force and superpowers, and you don't have a say because you are not in power—and quite frankly, many of you are not paying attention. From day to day, I notice many people living in their devices, paying absolutely no attention to what is going on around them. You are on your phones when you should be working, when you are eating, when walking in the park, and when driving. I am sure you are also on your phone when you are taking a poop. (Hope you have your cameras covered.)

What if your food were controlled? Your income? What if we were all set on the same income, amount of food, and healthcare? This is the direction we are going. When you become aware of what is happening, you can make a choice to pay attention, not participate, remove yourself from the situation, or stand up and decide not to allow it to happen. The only way the future can change is if the younger generations stand together and decide what they will and will not tolerate.

This means you may not be able to order something off Amazon and have it delivered to your door. As teenagers, we want cool stuff—cool clothes, cars, and gadgets; beauty, popularity, and success. We don't realize the impact of everything going on around us. None of this really matters when it comes down to it. What matters is your superpowers, super shifts, biofield, and life force. That is where the true power lies. Remember, you are a battery. Outside forces want to own, control, and manipulate that energy in their favor.

There is a very real possibility that you may have to live like the pioneers did, by surviving off the land and relying only on yourself for your well-being—living with less, living in freedom, and living off the grid and away from the digital matrix. When you buy into the digital matrix system, you are its life force slave. Is that what you want for your future? Never being able to reach your fullest potential? Missing your soul purpose destination? Selling off your soul?

I believe some of you may be figuring this out, which is why change has accelerated. You have been forced to believe, create, do, and become things you were never meant to, and it makes you feel . . . off. The time has come to get into your alignment.

We have the capability to live longer, healthier lives. We are conditioned to believe we are limited—in actuality, we are unlimited.

It took me a little while to put all the pieces together, but when I connected the dots, this is the feeling I got: smart cities will be powered by your super-powerful life force energy. So there would be no more classic cars with gas-powered engines, no freedom of choice, only one type of healthcare system offered, and only a certain amount of money allocated for people to live off of. Sounds like robotic automation with no freedom of choice. Are you ready to have your soul overtaken by AI robots?

You have been partially stunned into submission due to the digital matrix. *Snap out of it.* Put your devices down, look around, listen, and pay attention. If these ideas go into effect, this will take your freedom to travel; you wouldn't have the means or money to support it. Your healthcare would determine what you can and cannot do with your body. You have the option to work with incredible healers all over the world, thanks to the internet; so why is our healthcare system telling us we have to carry health insurance or pay the price?

We would be like animals in a cage with an invisible fence.

I have witnessed the city I live in change dramatically. I have noticed that basics such as food and gas have become so costly that we will eventually have no choice but to travel by bike or foot. Eventually it will become impossible for anyone to get out. We will be trapped in a mind-control system of living the way someone else wants us to.

What is important to you? Your freedom? Or your stuff?

## INFLUENCE

We see lots of propaganda these days. Propaganda is communication used to influence or persuade an audience to further an agenda; it may not be objective and may selectively present facts to encourage a particular outcome. Social media is being controlled, cut off, and limited as well, which is preventing freedom of the press. Assemblies are forming because there are people out there who want you to wake up, be aware, and know the truth. Humanity is becoming divided. Many of those who have been trained to fall in line have chosen not to take a stand. They don't want to cause waves or draw attention; after all, who wants the world's eyes on them?

Humans, you are being misled. It's a virtual reality takeover by artificial intelligence. Please wake up.

All I can say at this point is you must protect your superpowers, life force, super shifts, and your biofield. Get clear by removing toxins in your body, stop taking the digital matrix poison, get off the marijuana, stop drinking, stop the abuse, and stop the human trafficking. The world is changing, and we need to pay attention, take precautions, be intentional, and be very aware of what is coming next.

## TRANSHUMANISM

Now let's talk about transhumanism. This is beyond what a human being should ever become.

Are you ready to hear this? Transhumanism is when your body is augmented by technological advances. I am already seeing examples online in articles stating that llama blood may help with COVID. No way. There should be no mixing of our DNA with other sources. We need to stay holistically human. Outside forces are going to promise physical enhancement, expanded consciousness, machine embodiment, space travel adaptation, alien species embodiment, extended longevity, robotic embodiment, cloning, and psychosocial and emotional enhancement. We don't need any of this. Talk about psychologically jacking you up for eternity.

We have a life cycle for a reason. In fact, we could all could live close to 120 years and beyond if they didn't spend so much time trying to take us down and manipulate our genes. *Enough*. Transhumanism is a test. It's AI trying to hack your body, mind, and soul. You already have superpowers.

Have you seen the hand-scanning devices in the stores? And now they want to install a chip in our hands to pay for food and services, operate cars, and gain doorway access. Do not do this. This is all about stealing your life force energy—with your consent! AI will be able to read how you are thinking and feeling from the chip and then alter your life force however it chooses. Think about it: the moment you don't have any money for something, what is your body going to do? Move right into fear, giving them twice the amount of energy. They will completely own you.

This concept inspired me to learn about hand palmistry. And what I discovered is that the lines in your hands change as you gain experience. Be very careful about who looks at your hand, for the hand holds your soul's secrets. And it's not just the lines in your palm: it's the distance between your fingers, the curve of your hand, and the shape of your fingernails; and believe it or not, your fingers tie in to the planets. Palmistry is a science that can determine someone's destiny, psychology, and future. When you scan your hand, they know everything about you instantly. They know your genetic DNA imprint. Do not use an app on your phone to scan your hand for a palmistry reading.

## PHYSIOGNOMY, A.K.A. FACE READING, AND FINGERPRINTS

Do you know why your devices scan your face to be unlocked? AI reads you by the shape of your face and each area of your face: forehead, eyes, mouth, nose, lips, etc. It is using something called physiognomy, which is the art of getting a personality reading based on facial features. Do you know what the lines in your forehead are connected to? Planets. Notice a pattern here yet? Think about how AI could be using your face to determine who you are. Physiognomy covers parent relations, career/success, general life, love and emotion, and fertility. Even the color of our eyes gives away information about us.

Each person also has their own unique fingerprint—hence why our phones scan our thumbs to open the device. Our identity has been tracked, compiled, and filed away for quite some time.

## ADDICTED TO TECHNOLOGY

Younger generations need to come together and stand up to negative changes instead of hiding behind devices and unknowingly contributing to the illusion. AI is hijacking you. It will trickle down to your kids and grandkids. It will be the new normal, and then just normal to new humans brought into the world who don't know any other way. No matter how it's marketed, transhumanism will ruin humanity. You might notice doctors promoting it, too; even if those doctors don't agree with it, they'll want to keep their jobs. In fact, that happened with the COVID vaccine. Doctors were pushing it when they didn't even want it.

I urge you to research "The Elephant in the Room" on https://www.skirsch.com. Steve Kirsch provides 300 pages of slides documenting how the COVID vaccine has killed more people than the virus, is not good for anybody, and how nobody will talk or debate the topic when all the evidence and statistics back him up—yet another disturbing sign that whoever is running the show has zero concerns for humans. Please wake up if you are human, before you are not human.

Has anyone else noticed how all these new TV shows are addressing our current issues, trying to numb us to the fact that these so-called advancements are wrong for humanity? Netflix's movie *Spiderhead* addresses the testing of drugs on the human body and how people behave and react when given a dose of a certain drug. *Hello*. Human testing has been going on for years. There was even a particular drug in the *Spiderhead* film that got people to have sex with anyone who was sitting across from them, even if that particular individual opposed their values, beliefs, and ideas of a partner.

Check out *Upload* on Amazon Prime about the digital afterlife, which feels like a complete nightmare to me, as well as *Altered Carbon* on Netflix, where rich people can create an infinite number of clones and download their minds into them, essentially living forever. We are being exposed here to what could happen if this disrespect for our humanity continues.

## PORN AND DEHUMANIZATION

Online porn is a corrupt addiction to dehumanization. A friend told me of seeing porn on the internet where they could tell the woman was drugged; her soul had moved out of her body as she followed commands she didn't want to follow. In the end, my friend told me, they ended up crying from watching the disturbing interaction. I ask you: what the heck is going on here? Do you not see this or feel this?

Men will never be the same or know how to treat women properly due to this madness. I hear horror stories of men committing unacceptable acts because of watching too much porn. Showing women your private parts is not a turn-on but rather a forceful invitation that shows us you have no respect for us or yourself. I got flashed when I was a young woman after going to a fast food place late at night from a bar. The man approached us in a trench coat, opening it for us to view him. It's gross. These men seem to like the energetic reaction and get a high off of it, but clearly they are not thinking about how what they are doing will impact other people or make them feel. We don't want to see or be approached like that. It's uncomfortable, strange, and disturbing.

And women who dehumanize themselves through sexual solicitation are fools. They have a gazillion other choices, and there they go, selling their souls and life forces when those parts of them should be priceless.

This is not what we want to teach to our children. This is not what we want our children to see, witness, or become. We need to teach our children to become humans of honor.

## CRISPR

I heard about CRISPR at one of my coaching events. CRISPR is a gene-editing tool that allows researchers to easily alter DNA sequences and modify gene function. This offers a promise and hope to cure diseases. My take on this is mixed. I get a funny feeling when I read or watch anything on this subject; those are signs I tend to pay attention to—my intuition. Once again, someone is tampering with and altering our DNA, which has already pretty much been done with vaccines. In many cases, a lot of trial and error is required to create the magic concoction. And who is going to pony up to be the guinea pigs willingly? And what happens when the process goes in the wrong direction, maybe creating an entire new slew of problems and issues? All I can say is that altering your DNA should be carefully considered. Period.

## GEOENGINEERING

Believe it or not, our air, water, food, and resources have been poisoned for decades. Yes, decades. One day, I went outside and noticed all these trails in the sky that were not normally there. And I got this funny feeling. Like, *Wait a minute. That doesn't look or feel right. What is happening in the sky?* I went on Facebook, and someone had just so happened to post about the documentary *FrankenSkies*, and the filmmaker was being interviewed about geoengineering and chemtrails on a podcast. So I did the research, listened to the podcast, and watched the documentary. What the heck has been going on right in front of us all these decades without anyone questioning the validity? What gives anyone the right to decide what is best for humanity and Mother Nature without any input from society?

So I asked around. I would say one in ten people had an idea of what geoengineering is. And the people who knew about it were appalled and concerned. So, yes, I am going to talk about it and bring awareness since not enough people are doing that. Not only do we need to talk about it, but we also need to address it, and we need to stop it altogether.

Climate geoengineering refers to intervention in the earth's atmosphere, oceans, and soils with the aim of reducing the effects of climate change. What is geoengineering doing to humanity? What's happening to our air, water, and environment, the animals, and the earth is destroying all of us, but geoengineering is a misleading solution that aims to address the symptoms of climate change but ignores the true causes.

Planes fly above the earth and release chemicals into the air known as chemtrails. One day, I noticed microscopic shards of metals flying through the air, and that is when it hit me. No one can see it, unless you are vibrating at a very high frequency to access the energy field in the upper densities. That is why they don't understand it. We are breathing all those fine metals into our bodies, which is messing up our central nervous system, in addition to causing brain fog, leading to memory loss—hence all the elderly suffering from Alzheimer's disease; they have been breathing it in and eating it for decades. Metals are poison to the human body. The metals are falling to the earth, affecting our food and water, our homes. There is no escaping.

WTF, people. This is madness. Why are these things being allowed to continue unchallenged?

## 5G PROTECTION

Since the human body is made up of energy, we need to protect it. New products are hitting the market to combat 5G radiation in the energetic human body: special cell phone cases, blankets, clothing, hats, socks, and underwear are being created by those who are aware of how 5G is affecting the human population. Many people do not yet understand that we are being poisoned. You need to protect yourself. We need resources to combat the negative frequencies in order to help keep us aligned with ourselves.

I have a few items from https://www.ClimateCleaners.com that can protect you and your family. I have a antiradiation protector case over my Wi-Fi router and an EMF guard over the smart meter that tracks my household energy consumption. We really have to take precautions to protect ourselves now and in the future.

This chapter got a bit intense in the end. I don't say any of this to scare you. I am trying to inform you so you can outmaneuver the system. We all have been manipulated, programmed, persuaded, and drugged for a very long time. Go back and read the beginning of this chapter to remind yourself of the superpowers you have access to and the magnificent power you have to protect your life force, biofield, mind, body, and soul. You have an incredible opportunity to use the right tools, make the right choices, and live with intention and clarity. Life is an adventure of tests and trials. Humans are a superpower to be reckoned with.

You can learn more about the resources I have discovered and will continue to update on my website at https://www.LuminaryHealingCenter.com.

### JOURNAL: Chapter 4

1. Write down hobbies you would like to try.
2. What superpowers would you like to have?
3. What are the ways to ground yourself?
4. How you feel about the smart city concept?
5. What changes will you put into place to align yourself?

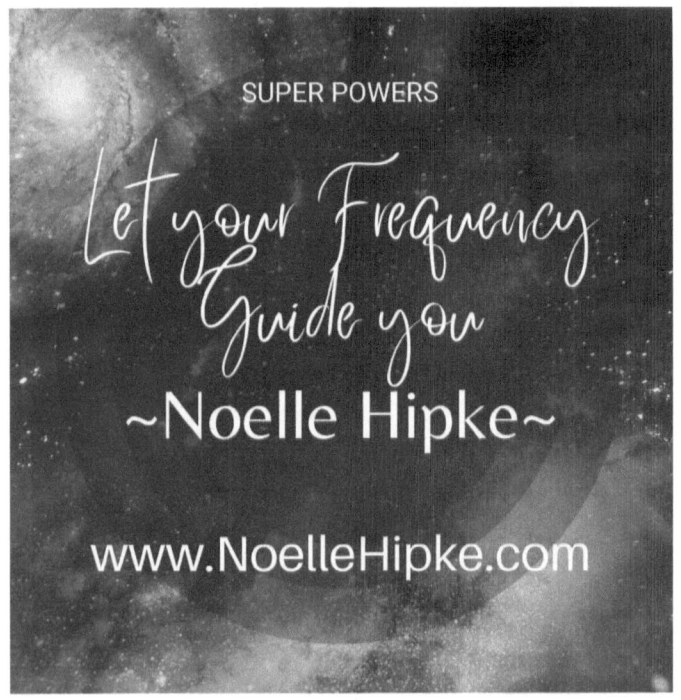

CHAPTER FIVE

# THE DIGITAL MATRIX IS TOXIC

Do you know what the best computer on earth is? Your brain. Your brain can easily be programmed by audio, visual, and subliminal messages—and I am sure by other forces we aren't even aware of. We are super-powerful beings, and there are multiple levels, realms, and dimensions that can be manipulated if we don't pay attention.

Think about it. We pull up a website, and the amount of blinking and flashing ads in the background can program our brain with whatever data someone wants to pop into our head.

5G is a frequency we can't hear, but it still affects our biology and cells. I know a lot of studies haven't surfaced yet on this topic, but that doesn't mean the effects don't exist. It hijacks our overall well-being. We all have devices, our kids have devices, and there are 5G towers everywhere. No one is feeling normal anymore, and we have to draw attention to it and change it right now.

## APPLICATIONS, A.K.A. APPS

Remember me telling you to always consider what other countries might be doing? Learn and listen. Other countries are making apps that track you and your data. If you put your birthday in, an address, or offer any personal information, assume that strangers have access to it and are reading it. Yep. There is no privacy anymore unless you only get a special phone and use it just for phone calls.

Likewise, every time you send someone a text, assume others are watching. Your data is not personal at all. You are being tracked, and your data is being used to influence and persuade you to do things. And some of those things may involve making bad choices. Outsiders are programming you how to think, act, and feel. That is why there is so much depression in the world. People feel terrible about themselves because of the toxic information being programed in their brains.

## PHONE ZOMBIES

I get phone calls with no one on the other end. What if vibrational frequencies that the human ear can't detect are being pushed out? We need to know about them so we can be aware. When I get a phone call with no one on the phone from a number I don't know, I hang up right away. I would say the safest bet is to only answer calls from people you know. That invisible vibrational frequency could be sending you messages to take your own life.

A lot of outside influences come in through texts, voicemails, and sound frequencies. Some of the phone calls and contacts made are false, trying to get you to believe a certain way so you behave a certain way. You cannot assume whoever is on the other end is normal and has good intentions. This is a wake-up call to put down your devices and turn to books, libraries, and other resources to get the info you need. Only use your phone for phone calls.

I say all this because I have been on the internet a very long time, and I have witnessed the difference between how I feel when I am on it and when I am not. There is a freedom of happiness when you control what goes into your mind. I control it by listening to audiobooks, podcasts, meditations, webinars, and seminars. I put on a booty bag (a.k.a. fanny pack) with an EMF phone protector and place wired headphones into my phone and leave my hands free to do things while I program my brain with what I want to feed it. Why wired headphones? Because wireless headphones carry a radiation frequency right to your brain when you put them in your ears. This can cause brain tumors, brain manipulation, brain function problems, and who knows what else.

I also got rid of my Apple Watch. That radiation-emitting tracking device was on me twenty-four seven, which is definitely not good for the body. These devices hijack the central nervous system and send our daily body activities and stats who knows where. See what I am getting at here? We have to think before we do things. Just because a product has creative, high-impact marketing doesn't mean we have to buy into it. I want you to start thinking, *Is this good for my body? What could happen if I allow this?*

Slight tangent: Start reading labels on the products you use. I recently bought some bath salts and forgot to read the label. They were from China, and a logo on the back stated it could cause cancer and reproductive harm. There is nothing natural about that, so I tossed the brand-new bag out.

So, back to podcasts, audiobooks, meditations, webinars, and seminars. I am in charge of how I feel. By controlling and monitoring how much info we let into our personal database system, we can be whomever we want.

I haven't listened or watched the news in twenty years. Some of the sickest people I know have the news constantly running in the background. Don't let this be you. And if your parents have it on, try to avoid it and get out of the room. It could be hard to convince them to put the media down since they have been programmed to watch it. News channels never report anything positive, and that negative energy affects you.

Ever have your ears ring? Messages from other frequencies are being sent to you. Sometimes it may mean you are transcending to a higher level in the field of life—or you could be getting a download of information that is transmitting coded information to the brain, storing the data in your cellular memory to use as needed. It could also be sending the message you are going down a level—if you aren't taking care of yourself—as a reminder to pay attention.

When you are tapped into your superpowers, you are tapped into your own database and not someone else's. It takes a bit of work in this day and age with all the wireless devices spinning madly around us. Honestly, the best thing to do is disconnect. I know you might not want to hear this, but put your phone away for most of the day and only check it once in a while as a trial start. Let's say that at the top of every hour, you go and check it and give yourself five minutes or less. Place it in a cabinet away from where you will be. You don't want a device that is emitting radiation right up against your body all the time. And if you are constantly holding it, what do you think the energy from the device is doing to your hands? Think future arthritis and hand pain. No one wants that.

You have to get used to living without it. We have become so codependent on devices that give us nothing in return but a buzz in our head that makes us not feel good about ourselves. Your friends can wait. And if you tell them what you are doing, you all will know to check your phones at the top of the hour to connect. But the best way to connect is in person. Screw all these so-called smart devices. It has made people so dumb. We don't even know how to have real conversations in person, nor do we want to conduct business in person. When I meet people these days, I ask them to turn off their phone. I don't want anything to do with their phones, just them.

I woke up at 4:28 a.m. to write this piece; that is when my higher self is most clear. Why? Because I have just slept and cleared my head of all media input and I am in alignment with myself. I have detoxified my body, and clarity really starts to set in.

When you are clean and clear is when your superpowers appear.

Get off the net. It is ruining our lives and sucking your soul out of you. I know you have felt it, or you wouldn't be human. You just haven't been able to identify it yet. And that is exactly what I am here to do. I can identify it because I am clean, clear, and I can recall what life was like when we didn't have it. We didn't have all the mental and emotional problems we do today. It was so much easier, fun, happy, and interactive, and the positive energy we shared with one another was amplified. We would play games, go to the park, hit the beach, go shopping, go out to lunch, ride bikes, play sports, read books, bake, create, and the list is endless.

The internet is limiting you. You are unlimited and unstoppable when you control outside forces. You can create your own force field and maintain your biofield by paying attention. Your life force is worth more than money. Money is stealing our energy because we give it value. What if money suddenly didn't have any value? Then what is important? Good food? Health? Remember, we don't really need all that crap we buy; it loads us down and prevents us from roaming around in a wonderful free world. Self-care, hobbies, activities, travel, and nature are the real fun of life.

It is time to disconnect and monitor ourselves and each other. Be accountable for these life-sucking devices and prevent them from constantly interrupting your wonderful life. Life without interruptions and radiation frees you to gain access to your superpowers.

## DNA AND ANCESTRY WEBSITES

There are toxins being put into the body, manipulating your DNA and your mind. Altering your DNA could affect the children you have in the future or your fertility.

What I have learned about DNA is that our bodies can recover and realign when treated properly and given the right conditions. It may take some work and not happen overnight, but we are working on that. Your DNA will guide you on what to do for you. A lot of cool things are in your lineage genes. What if someone in your timeline thousands of years ago was a warrior? There is a good chance you have a bit of warrior in you. They may have fought with swords, ridden horses, and shot bows or guns. You may have really good aim and be good at sports, all because of the genes in your body and heritage. You activate them in a less lethal way as you practice and play. You do it energetically instead of "to the death."

Many people try to learn about their DNA lineage through ancestry testing. You might think these sites are simply helping you find information about your DNA and past relatives. Think again. This is a massive database with your private information. Do you want other countries, companies, and people to know what your bloodline contains? What if someone needed a particular body part and you had the perfect DNA match? What if you had royalty in your bloodline? What if these companies could tell what ailments might affect your health by looking at your DNA—and then trigger them?

Do you know how much this massive database is worth today? From what I can gather, it looks to be over five billion dollars, with more than thirty billion online records and more than twenty million people using the DNA network.

Why do you think that is? Why would your DNA be worth so much? Do you think healthcare companies might be interested in getting their hands on this data? Do you think other countries would want to look at this for biological warfare? Biological warfare, also known as germ warfare, uses biological toxins or infectious agents such as bacteria, viruses, insects, and fungi with the intent to kill, harm, or incapacitate humans, animals, or plants as an act of war. Biological weapons are living organisms or replicating entities.

So I ask you: are you paying attention to what you are offering up to companies, apps, programs, and people you don't know? There is no such thing as privacy anymore.

## DIGITAL MATRIX

I have witnessed people suffering from PTSD and other mental issues due to vaccines, the internet, abuse in the home, an unhealthy work environment, and the list goes on. This is what causes sickness in the body: being stuck in unhealthy states for a long period of time. And you need to learn how to snap out of it mentally, emotionally, and physically. This is not easy for some of us, especially if you are sensitive.

Some humans think and feel more deeply than others, and it can take some time to get realigned if we don't learn how to snap out of it.

I left a job that required me to work on the internet eight hours a day. And when I walked away, it became very clear that the people I worked with were angry, abusive messes due to stress. I was in a part of the digital matrix I desperately needed to get out of; it was sucking the life force right out of me.

It is time to protect ourselves, families, friends, and children by monitoring the digital matrix. We have to prevent it from entering into our field, bombarding us with unsolicited information.

There are bad people trolling for what they can take from you: your identification, sex, mind, body, organs, energy, life force, and soul. It's really important you take this information into consideration and do something about it. Right now. You are not free. You are an energetic slave being programmed like a massive human database. You have an amazing power source of energy right within you: your soul. It is what guides you.

For decades I have been told what to believe, how to behave, and what to do. And I did many of those things against what my gut was telling me. Why? Because everyone else I was surrounded by was pushing their energy on me to do this or that. But once you gain control of your own power source and realize the power of your soul to guide you and that don't need anyone else, you have activated your superpowers.

When I activated my superpowers, I discovered that people who no longer aligned with my high vibration fell away, and I was completely okay with that because I was more powerful making my own choices than listening to their mumbo-jumbo. All the answers lie within. That is what your higher self is for—to guide you to what is right for you. I can't tell you how many times I didn't listen to my higher self when I was younger, and I still sometimes make that mistake. But I guarantee you, it's always right. By being clear, clean, and clever, you can turn on your superpowers and become the power source you are meant to be for yourself, your community, your company, for humanity. You are so stinking powerful that you are unlimited. Endless. Infinite.

Our bodies don't have to age. We don't have to have sickness. When you're ready, dive in and do the work. When you work with and heal your soul, you heal the past, as well as the present and future generations in your timeline. How powerful it that? The power lies within you to change human history and existence for the better. This is exactly why I am writing this book. My goal in this life has always been to heal the soul, and now, by divine guidance, I am sharing how to do just that.

The secret is to have compassion, forgiveness, and unconditional love for one another, no matter what. Take care of your body, mind, and soul so your mind cannot get hijacked. When people vibrate low, you can feel it by the way they make you feel energetically, how they act, believe, and behave. Know they have been hijacked and forgive them, for they do not know. Focus on health and happiness. Once you get these in alignment, heal your wounds and traumas, and break through your fears and barriers, you elevate and transcend to a very high vibrational frequency of love. Once you gain purity of compassion for all others no matter what they do or how badly they treat you, and once you forgive everyone in your life for their mistakes/mistreatment and offer them unconditional love no matter what the circumstances, you become one with the universe. You become pure light. In the end, we all become one together.

Wowee. Did I just write that? I got chills all over my body. This is what happens when you are aligned and fulfilling your higher needs or prophecy. Get out of the digital matrix, and you will have a life that you can define through your own choices and behaviors. Other people who are constantly on their devices will never vibrate at the same level. And you may have to let them go.

You are being called to rise above and remove yourself from this addiction. It is a test to see if you can overcome, outsmart, and outmaneuver the game of life. If you think outsiders are not using your camera, audio, and mind to monitor you, think again. Neuromarketing telepathy is being used here through AI and your devices. You have been programmed to believe that having the latest device is needed, but having the latest gadget isn't cool anymore—getting rid of it is. You have the power to remove the toxicity from your life.

Those devices are getting more and more advanced with every upgrade of mind control and telepathy mechanisms. Don't let them derail you. No one can tell you how to achieve your dreams. You are a trailblazer creating your own path, and you already have the answers of the universe within you. No college, no parent, no friend will ever know your superpowers unless you choose to share them with the world on your own terms. Get off the digital matrix and remove their power source: you. You are a field of energy being used like a battery.

You will never need any of the crap you buy. In fact, one day you will be looking to either throw it in the trash, give it away, or donate it. What has value is your body, mind, and soul. This is what you need to feed and take care of the most.

Build your own community of people who share the same values. Live off the land, respect nature, and retain heritage by pulling in wisdom from elders before it is lost forever. Love and appreciate one another, for Mother Nature will provide to those who love, respect, and appreciate the wisdom and guidance she has to offer.

Think about the Indians. They were here long before we took over their land, living off Mother Nature's bounty with values, morals, traditions, respect, and guidance from their elders. We need to go back to these roots, understand their strategies and traditions, look at other cultures to see what has worked in the past, and recreate our own new-world lives.

• • •

## TEXTING

I think texting is one of the biggest time and energy wasters today. When I was online dating, it seems like men wanted me to text my life through the phone. It is one of the most dangerous and dead-end situations anyone could subject themselves to. There is no personalization this way, just information. This is not a form of good communication. It is riddled with misunderstandings and misrepresentation. Nobody needs to communicate like this unless they are a robot.

And why would anyone in their right mind want to share their life story through text with someone they don't know? A text anyone could be reading, for that matter. You could be texting a robot, sending information to a database that is tracking your life story to take you down. "There is *no privacy*," I yell at you. So don't make the mistake of doing this. We are human beings in need of proper human interaction.

If the person avoids getting to know you personally and energetically, move on and let them go.

## Ghosting

Which brings me to the subject of ghosting—completely cutting contact with a person without warning or explanation. We never had this when I was a kid, but even adults ghost. Talk about immaturity. Someone who ghosts you is not worth your time or energy. Instead of saying, "Hey there, I have this going on" or "I am moving in another direction and I wish you well," they just stop responding to you. Which leaves you feeling confused, conflicted, rejected, and like you are unworthy.

If they don't respond to the first text, give them a break. We all forget sometimes or don't have the time or mindset to respond the proper way. But if you send more than three texts in a reasonable time frame and don't get a response, run away. This is not at all how you deserve to be treated. You don't want to set the tone that you will tolerate this behavior; they will continue to take you on this emotional roller coaster as long as you stay on. I don't want you to get upset about it, either. I want you to realize that the issue is with them, not you. Take your superpower life force energy back and keep it to yourself. No one truly deserves it but you, and if they can't reciprocate, they don't deserve you.

• • •

## GASLIGHTING

I once dated a guy who was an expert at gaslighting. He drove me crazy—at least, that was the way he made me feel. If someone is gaslighting you, they act as if your feelings are wrong, don't acknowledge your needs and make you feel wrong for having them, and deny facts and energies you feel. It's an expert form of manipulation. I remember telling him I felt funny. My body read his energy and felt something was off. I mentioned I thought he wasn't really where he told me he had been for the last few hours. He proceeded to yell at me, belittle me, distract me, argue with me, put me down over and over, and deny he was doing anything wrong. He turned the argument around, saying I was the one causing the trust issue.

However, my higher self was telling me something different. My body was shaking and felt completely off. When I told him this, he acted even more frustrated and grew very angry. Later I discovered he was seeing another woman, whom I had introduced him to. Talk about betrayal and lies. Energy does not lie.

Gaslighting can have long-term effects psychologically, emotionally, and physically, and I felt all the symptoms from his abuse. Gaslighting turns the victim's emotions, awareness, and who they are as people against them. So when you feel off, question your environment and those around you. Separate yourself so you can hear your higher self and get into alignment. This is how you know what is right for you.

## ARTIFICIAL INTELLIGENCE

I recently watched a show called *A.rtificial I.mmortality*. One segment is about artificially intelligent clones that move, behave, react, and look like real human beings. In due time, we may have a hard time telling the difference between a real human and these AI robot clones. In fact, there is a very good chance they are already integrated into society—yet another deceit to wrap our heads around.

The premise of another segment is that the human soul is capturable data. In order to create an avatar in the digital matrix using this capturable data, you would upload all your memories via photos, videos, and pages of personal information. The show claims we have already given away and consented to sharing all our personal data by participating in online social media platforms. It goes on to say that now and in the future, we will want to guard our personal information and only grant access to an exclusive group. The particular company highlighted by the show goes to extreme measures to ensure people's data is put into the right hands and secured.

In one example, a fifty-two-year-old mother uploads all of her personal data with this company in order to share it exclusively with her family when she is no longer physically here on this planet. When the kids interact with their avatar mother on the screen, they feel the avatar doesn't have a soul. I think it's rather creepy. This new AI concept is a bit hard to digest at first; we are being introduced to AI clones. However, after processing the information, I discovered a new perspective that I want you to think about.

We are all light energy. What if when we pass away, that light energy is harvested and hosted by the digital matrix for eternity? We could be cloned or transferred into a robotic body and captured forever. How is that for thinking outside the stratosphere? No one would have to physically age, opting instead to live on forever in a robotic body.

The kids feel the mom's avatar doesn't have a soul, which makes it feel flat and purely data based. Of course, the mom is still alive and her soul is still in her current body. What would happen if she passes and her soul moves out of the body? If the soul is freed from the body to roam, she should be able to go wherever she chooses, right? However, if the light being's soul is captured before it can ascend, the soul could become an eternal slave, loaded into a robotic body driven by the digital matrix.

Would you consider this option to have immortality? Would you want to interact with these avatars? We could replicate famous educated people, leaders, or whomever anyone deemed worthy of controlling the world.

Let's face it, not everyone out there is working for the good of mankind. If your file got hacked or put in the wrong hands, the situation could very well be taken to an extreme level we may not have considered. What if someone wanted to clone you and sell you to others as a companion? I have to admit, as a single woman, it's appealing to imagine the ability to pick a man who is exactly what I want—one who stimulates me intellectually, emotionally, and mentally while also helping with household chores. He would have no ego and accept and allow me to be authentically me. Eventually he could turn into my caregiver should I need it as I grow older.

But if we can't tell the difference between a human and a robot, what do you think that would do to society?

So, I present this information as something for you to consider and process as I do the same. I see both sides of the coin and will sit on the sidelines for a while to witness what becomes of it. In the meantime, be cautious.

## TRIPODS BOOK SERIES

In 1981, I was in the sixth grade. Our teacher read to the class a book series written by John Cristopher about beings called Tripods: *The White Mountains* (1967), *The City of Gold and Lead*, and *The Pool of Fire* (1968).

That series had a profound impact on me at that time and still does to this day.

This science fiction series was rather surreal and in my eyes could very well be happening today. The premise involves humanity being enslaved by an alien race called the Masters, who use Tripods—gigantic, three-legged machines that walk the face of the earth—to overtake humanity. These aliens control humans by implanting a metal "cap" on their heads at the age of fourteen that suppresses free will and individuality, enslaving the humans to serve the Masters. This complete mind control sounds pretty much like what our digital matrix is doing to human society today, only without the "caps." Tracking devices are implanted in the humans, which I would say currently aligns with the apps on our cell phones. Humans who aren't capped join the resistance and flee to the White Mountains to live freely.

A regional sporting event is hosted to find the strongest boys in the world, and the winners are taken to the Tripod city. The city is under a gigantic dome astride a river. Beautiful females are terminated and preserved for the Masters to adore, and the males are kept as slaves. The city creates artificial green air for the Masters to breathe, creating a heavy gravitational pull. The boy slaves need breathing masks in order to survive, making it hard to move freely, and people age rather quickly due to the heavy gravitational pull—hence the need for young and strong boys. Several boys realize the implications and strategize to save their world from the aliens. One Master reveals a plan to replace Earth's atmosphere with the Masters' toxic air to enable full control of the planet—for he who controls the weather, air, and environment controls the planet, which still holds true to this day.

The boys manage to escape the Tripod city and organize an uprising. They discover ways to attack, overtake the Masters within the city, and force open the airlocks, exposing aliens to the atmosphere, which kills them instantly. Several attacks are undertaken—some successful, some not. Some sacrifice their lives and become heroes. The boys regain the planet. Eventually, the Masters' spaceship returns to destroy the remaining alien cities in order to stop the human race from reverse-engineering their technology.

A prequel of the series came twenty years later, called *When the Tripods Came* (1988). Now, I haven't read this book yet, but when I do the research, it sounds eerily similar to what could be happening in the digital matrix today. Unable to beat humanity and concerned that human technology might overtake the Masters, the aliens hypnotize humans through a television program that causes mania (which sounds like video games to me), in the end ultimately overtaking the humans and beginning the metal "capping" process.

It is all about being invaded and enslaved. You can't see it, put a finger on it, or define it unless you have the knowledge to connect the invisible dots and take a distant perspective. I don't say this to scare anyone; I share this to give you accelerated clarity on what I see, feel, and have witnessed in my lifetime.

I suggest you seek out the Tripods book collection or the BBC television series *The Tripods*. I find it interesting that this particular series focuses on beings made of pure energy. This brings me back to my feeling that smart cities are designed to take control of your life force energy. Interestingly enough, I put the smart-cities piece together first and then weeks later recalled the Tripods trilogy, did the research, and was stunned to notice the similarities.

There are moments I am blown away by the knowledge flowing through me and the information I can pull out from decades-old memories. Once again, I am being divinely guided to present what I have learned on my journey and give you the resources to determine what is taking place in the world and how you would like to move through life from here.

. . .

## IN CLOSING

This is so powerful that I had to write it again at the end of this chapter because sometimes we have to hear and read things multiple times. Please consider saying it out loud so you can hear it in your own voice.

The secret is to have compassion, forgiveness, and unconditional love for one another, no matter what. Take care of your body, mind, and soul so your mind cannot get hijacked. When people vibrate low, you can feel it by the way they make you feel energetically and how they act, believe, and behave. Know they have been hijacked and forgive them, for they do not know. Focus on health and happiness. Once you get these in alignment, heal your wounds and traumas, and break through your fears and barriers, you transcend to a very high-vibrational frequency of love. Once you become compassionate for all others no matter what they do or how badly they treat you, and once you forgive everyone in your life for their mistakes/mistreatment and offer them unconditional love no matter what the circumstances, you become one with the universe. You become pure light. You become infinite, endless, and unlimited. In the end, we all become one together.

### JOURNAL: Chapter 5

1. What you would put your energy into if money had no value?
2. What would you choose to do with your time and energy if there were no internet?
3. Are there any apps you should remove from your devices?
4. What new perspectives has this chapter on the digital matrix made you think about?

Gratitude Journal: Make sure you are writing daily in your gratitude journal. It will help you keep your eyes on what matters most and bring you into alignment with your higher self and good vibrations.

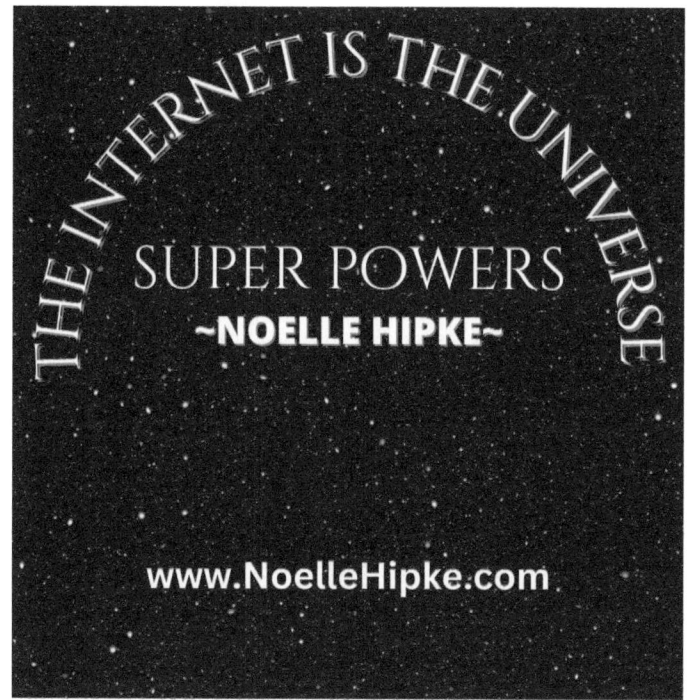

## CHAPTER SIX

# EMOTIONAL INTELLIGENCE

Emotional intelligence, or EI, is something we should be teaching kids from a young age. So I have devoted an entire section to this topic. I have worked with many people with horrible EI, and it negatively impacts the work environment. This trait is one you should want to master and acquire at any age.

Organizations hire and promote based on emotional intelligence, not based on certain skills or intelligence quotients (IQ). EI is the ability to understand and express emotions while using empathy when communicating with others, and it ignites key factors that set high-performing individuals apart from the rest of the crowd. EI skills work well in your workplace, school systems, personal life, and when navigating the digital matrix. EI can help you reach your goals or stack a winning team. Mastering your EI will amplify positive relationships with others, which in turn helps you build collaborative projects that can impact the world. EI is one of the top evolving skills you need to develop and master in this lifetime.

You can tap into your superpowers by growing, enhancing, and developing your emotional intelligence. Remember, you also need to detox, drink living water, and eat right in order to tap in, which will have a direct impact on your achievements, relationships, and performance. Learn it and practice it, just like with anything else you want to be good at. This is how you change your body—with repetition.

When we pay attention, we can catch ourselves and notice when others are trying to manipulate us. EI also utilizes IQ and personality.

When you have them all working in harmony, it is much easier to identify when things are out of sorts, solve problems, and make good decisions.

There are four areas of EQ: self-awareness, self-management, social awareness, and relationship development—how we make other people feel, how we feel, and how we all feel as a whole in conscious oneness. Look inward to focus on yourself and understand your emotions. A poor reaction to a situation often results from being triggered by a previous trauma that may be resurfacing. Learning to identify and manage this is key. Sometimes we don't see the issue until after the fact, days or hours later, but the whole idea of being aware, acknowledging, and redirecting yourself is what is important here. As you practice, you will notice, redirect, and master yourself. You can't control how others behave and respond; you can only control yourself.

In real estate, I learned to not make decisions quickly and told people not to take action until they had slept on the information overnight. Moving through the costs, inspections, repairs, financing, uncertainty, etc., is a very emotional process. Many people just wanted the upper hand. However, the best approach is to create a win-win situation for everyone. That way, no one feels discredited, and the transaction runs smoother. After cooling off, we were typically able to offer multiple solutions to get everyone on the same page. I've represented both the buyer and seller in several transactions, and this is the approach I found to be most effective. If you are hot and bothered by a situation, walk away. If you change the energy flow and regain your own alignment, clarity regarding next steps will come.

How do you think and react to situations? Emotions come in response to circumstances, so you can see why environment and energy exchange is very critical here. Emotions can be extreme or mild. What might really bother you one day might not the next. Drugs, unknowns, stress, and fear tamper with our nervous system, creating chaos in the body. Detoxing the body, avoiding drugs/alcohol and stressful situations, and living our life in faith over fear empowers us to own and switch on our superpowers.

Our emotions help us judge and assess a situation. They can also cause a physical response, such as shaking or sweating. How we interact with one another based on how we assess the situation is a behavioral reaction. It is important you pay attention and listen to your body when you get worked up. It is sending you signals of fight, flight, or freeze.

## WHAT IS THE FIGHT-FLIGHT-FREEZE REACTION?

The fight-flight-freeze is an automatic physiological reaction to an event that is perceived as stressful or frightening. The perception of a threat triggers the sympathetic nervous system and activates the stress response that prepares the body to fight, flee, or freeze. These are survival skills. Think of how animals react when their lives are threatened.

Notice how your body reacts in certain situations. Does it tense up?

When you notice your body taking on the fight-flight-freeze response . . .

1. Listen up
2. Pause
3. Evaluate
4. Reset

• • •

## STRESS

### At Work

Many of us have worked in stressful environments. In addition, many people unexpectedly had to work from home during the pandemic. When starting any new position, working from home forces you to learn on the job through email or Zoom calls instead of in-person, on-the-job training. Only 10 percent of the population learns through reading, so obtaining information days later, often through email, makes it difficult to retain.

I am sure many of you have suffered as a consequence of drastic changes until you found your balance. Some of us enter fight-flight-freeze modes in response. Our bodies can react to the oxidative stress with body shakes, heart palpitations, sleep deprivation, and aches. Paralyzed by fear of the unknown, our concentration levels can diminish. It can create a horrible, toxic cycle if we are not paying attention.

Single moms have to tolerate a lot in order to keep a job to pay the bills and take care of their children. At one point in my life, I grew suicidal, stuck in an unhealthy loop I saw no way out of. All I wanted to do was make it stop. During the week of Christmas, my daughter walked into my bedroom to find me on the floor on my hands and knees, crying uncontrollably. At that moment, the reasons for suicide became clear to me. My soul was dying; it wanted out, and that was when I knew my body was trying to tell me something. It was trying to tell me I was not in alignment with myself. My job was killing my self-worth and self-esteem. It was affecting all the cells in my body, which created extreme stress. That is when I researched stress and learned about oxidative stress.

## Oxidative Stress

Did you know oxidative stress can cause accelerated aging? That is one reason why some people the same age look totally different. Subjecting one's body to bad foods, drugs, stress, lack of sleep, etc., over years can take a toll. The cells in your body respond to everything.

I could perform the job, but there were invisible forces working behind the scenes. I had to take some days off to clear my head to understand that I was in a no-win situation. I'd spent about $13,000 in a two-month period, trying many of the healing modalities I am sharing with you in this book. And get this: not one of them was going to work unless I completely removed myself from the toxic work situation. We can't control or change how others think or behave. I felt energetically drained, so it was time to go.

When you get to this point in your life, that should push you to realize you are not in alignment with who you are and what you are here to do on this planet.

I suffered for many months and my health took a hit before I was able to identify that the environment was not good for me and to remove myself from a situation that was not healthy for my personal progress. I want to empower you with this knowledge so you and your body will know how to hear and understand what is right for you. You are going to face all kinds of situations on your journey, and once you know how to identify and assess, you have turned on your superpowers.

Believe me, you will face some very uncomfortable choices and scenarios, but that is how you grow and learn to align. Creating a supportive win-win situation is the name of the game.

## Public Speaking

For some reason, I can pull off public speaking and give detailed explanations on complex topics to people on all levels. It's one of my superpowers. I have learned this is in my DNA, thanks to Human Design. I believe my cells sense other people's energy and vibrations, and my body adjusts to accommodate their senses.

I don't always practice before presentations and videos, but doing them consistently is like using a muscle over and over; you tend to get naturally good at it. In order to present authenticity, you must be genuine and not sound like you are just presenting facts. I usually jot down a list of items I want to talk about and dive in. You must project an energy, a vibration that draws the audience in, and use verbiage that compels them to listen and learn more. Your voice, body language, and actions all play a part and sometimes are more important than what you are saying. People read your energy, enthusiasm, passion, and projection.

However, you might feel a lot of stress with public speaking, leading to fear, anger, and sweaty palms when standing in front of a room of people. I remember having to go to the front of the room from time to time in school. What I learned is to prepare. Prepare your presentation, practice in front of the mirror, or film yourself. This way you can look at your body language, hear how you project your voice, and make alterations to your performance. How do you want to present yourself?

My advice to you is relax, let go, be who you are, and just flow. If you don't get it perfect, so what? Nobody is perfect, unless you are a programmed robot. All people are looking for is good entertainment. Throw something personal in there about what you learned or what you did or didn't like. This lets people know you are thinking, experiencing, learning, and interacting with them. You will impress the audience, teachers, and crowd when you perform off the cuff. If you trip, play into it; break out in a dance. Why not? They will never forget how well you handled yourself in a sticky situation. Bring them into the action and performance.

How you feel about the situation is important. People will feel the message you are projecting. Emotional intelligence drives your reactions, your attitude toward challenges, and your relationships. Do not react automatically. Manage how you behave, and the best way to do this is to pay attention, be clear (no drugs/alcohol), and stay self-aware. Emotional responses are so quick that it takes conscious practice to become aware of the process. Once you understand the automatic response, you can intercept and redirect the process and then make changes and alterations to your behaviors.

We often behave and think quickly, emotionally, and intuitively. Reshape the process by slowing down your thinking and being more deliberate and logical in the judgment call. By interpreting situations for what they really are and not acting from a place of emotions, you change the model.

Recognizing your emotions, responses, and reactions is the first step. Redirecting it is the next step. These are what I call R to the tenth power:

1. Remodel
2. Redesign
3. Reform
4. Reengineer
5. Restyle
6. Reformat
7. Rewrite
8. Reshape
9. Recast
10. Restructure

Any way you look at it, you are changing the patterns. It takes time and energy to bring your attention inward so you can alter your course. Remember, you can't control other people; you can only control you. You are using your superpowers when you are in complete control of your actions, thoughts, and emotions.

• • •

## TAKE CONTROL

To take control, you must accept your emotions and slow down your reactions.

We can't change what happened in the past, but we can learn from our experiences to change the present and future. This is exactly what the journey of life is all about: accumulation of experiences, lessons learned, successes, and failures. Emotions dictate our experience and how we function. In the heat of the moment, you may react poorly before you think. Forgive yourself and give yourself permission to be imperfect. Make a mental note, apologize if you have to, and make an extra effort to not let that happen again.

You must intercept the thoughts, feeling, and emotions created by the instigating event before they lead to behavior response. This takes practice. Take a moment to pause and assess the situation before you react. Excuse yourself to go to the bathroom, take a walk, dance, or do some deep breathing. Move the energy. Disrupt your emotional responses. Redirecting is the best action to take.

Personal reflection is a key part to understanding your patterns. You want to pay attention to trigger events or thoughts that consistently take you in the wrong direction. Be a detective and analyze your past responses.

## Being in Flow

When you are completely immersed in an activity, other distractions fade into the background. I literally shut myself off from the world when I want to accomplish anything on a grand scale. When you relax and get into flow, the universe will line up to put success in your path.

Flow happens to me when I write things like this book. I put my phone on mute and let divine guidance flow out through me and onto the pages. Sometimes I can't type fast enough, and I type eighty-five words per minute. Activities that give you flow will stretch you to evolve, feel effortless, and be rewarding. Sometimes after writing in this book I think, *Holy smokes. That sounds so good that I can't believe I wrote that. Thanks, universe, for helping me translate a great message.*

The benefits of energy flow include achieving peak performance, which activates your superpowers.

Focus on what you are good at, and capitalize on that. It will make you light up. Emotionally working in the energetic state of flow creates a positive mental experience. I learned to follow the flow of energy, and my life changed dramatically. It's a matter of aligning and not resisting. Resistance sabotages us. Clarify what "lights you up," which will get you into flow in your working/student/daily life. This helps you face challenges with confidence and build your self-esteem. You will just feel right. Finding and working with flow will help you build emotional intelligence and reengineer how you react to challenges and live your life. If you let everything else go, new information floods in, giving you the advantage.

## Stressful Situations

Let's face it: we are all going to encounter stressful situations on our journey. These situations tend to trigger us to react in the heat of the moment. So the goal is to break the chain reactions. It takes practice to do this. We will mess up many times, so don't beat yourself up. Eventually you will catch the triggers because you are aware and considering better options.

Here are a few ideas on how to gain control:

- Identify the emotional reactions you are having.
- Remove yourself from the situation and take deep breaths.
- Give yourself time to recover and step away from the energy cycle.
- Focus on feeling balanced emotionally and physically; take a walk to clear your head, or step into the bathroom to change a pattern frequency.
- Think about how you can achieve the results you want; use guided imagery or visualizations.
- Methodically choose how you will respond.

Make shifting perspective a way of life:

- Seek out different points of views.
- Ask more questions, and listen. Listen to what your body is telling you.
- Meet new people to build new healthy relationships and create new patterns.
- Read books on a variety of topics to grow and evolve.
- Listen to podcasts on topics you want to learn more about.

• • •

## IMPORTANT EI QUALITIES

1. Social awareness: the ability to understand others and respond to their needs and feelings. You apply social awareness to the world around you to create collaborative and successful relationships.
2. Self-awareness: looking inward to understand what is going on in your body and head.
3. Senses: Use your senses to gather information. Pay attention to details. Many of the details may be invisible or show through vibration, energy, color, body language, voice control, verbal tones. This helps you understand other people's thoughts and emotions, building your intuitive sense. Take notice of the information. Do you pick up on other people's social cues? How are they coming across?
4. Empathy: the ability to sense others' emotions, thoughts, and feelings. Can you put yourself in someone else's shoes? In their head?

### Empathy

I once went on a couple of dates with a man who told me his therapist said he could not feel empathy. Looking back, I can think of several humans who seemed to lack this trait altogether. When someone can't feel empathy, they can't understand you, sense you, or accept you, nor will they ever. This must be a very hard trait to live without. You go through life ignoring everyone else's needs and being unlikeable, driven solely by your own judgment and needs. So I urge you to think about being in someone else's shoes. We never really know what other people are going through, but sometimes if we align with them, we can sense them and their emotions. Do not assume you know exactly what a situation is like for someone else.

The goal is to give everyone compassion, forgiveness, and understanding. So display no judgment, only unconditional love.

Ways to develop empathy:

- Ask questions.
- Imagine how the other person may be feeling.
- Don't compare.
- Offer support.

Let the other person know you care and understand. A class I once took mentioned responding with "Thank you for sharing this with me" or "I don't know what to say. I am just glad you told me" to anything sensitive someone shares with you when you are not really sure what to say. It gives them acknowledgment and acceptance by offering support without a reaction. Often times, people just want to be heard and accepted.

## Communication

Communication involves getting your message out while gathering information from others. Most of what we communicate is unconscious and driven by our thoughts, feelings, and mood. Words, tone, and body language play as big a part as message, vibration, and energy. Listen. Being able to listen and observe is a superpower. A lot is being communicated when nothing is being said. Do you listen? How can you listen better?

## Nonverbal Communication

Many people can lie with their mouths, but their body is going to tell you the truth of the matter. Since we are all doing video calls these days, reading each other's body language is crucial to determining how well we are receiving one another.

Here are a few tips I wrote down when taking a class on nonverbal communication:

- Use hand gestures.
- Smile, be enthusiastic and engaging, and make eye contact.
- Be warm, friendly, and empathetic.
- Ask questions.
- Remember important details.
- Mirror and match others.
- Have self-awareness, self-control, and awareness of others.
- Speak slowly.
- Don't act defensive.
- Slow down your responses.
- Offer support.
- Listen, listen, listen.
- Observe.
- Hear what someone is saying.
- Emotion is information in motion.
- Do not cross arms, lean away, rub or wring hands, touch face, touch stomach.
- Think, *How am I coming across?*

. . .

## GETTING INTO STATE OF MIND

I find the best way to get in alignment with my higher self is to do things that make me really happy. And I do it intentionally. The goal is to get the cells in my body tingling. Then I am in the state of mind to do anything. I feel invincible.

Ways to get into state:
- Dance
- Sing
- Jump
- Yell
- Laugh
- Smile
- Play music
- Exercise

When I do this, I am lifting up my vibrational frequencies to higher levels in a process called leveling up.

## Level Up

When you level up, you energize the cells in the body to align to higher frequencies. By creating a pulsating rhythm, leveling up moves energy through the body and into higher realms of universal energy flow. Vibrating higher leads to a frequency upgrade, and your intuition will become stronger. Don't be alarmed when you notice how much other people's energy affects you. Other people's energy is often lower, which can drag you down. You may find you don't want to put your energy toward these people when you become attuned to your superpowers.

• • •

# RELATIONSHIP STRENGTHS

Utilize your unique style to generate connections and trust. This is what I call being authentic. Some people are blessed with charisma, yes. But all you have to do is call attention to yourself, pay attention, and modify yourself.

- Listen closely to others and watch for cues.
- Ensure people feel comfortable with the vibration.
- Pick up on group dynamics and energies.
- Make authentic eye-to-eye connections.
- Communicate clearly and precisely.

∙ ∙ ∙

## IN CLOSING

How do you think others perceive you? Do you understand what others are feeling and needing? Undertake the following to become more aware and level up your emotional intelligence:

1. *Review* how you manage your relationships. Look for areas to improve. We all have them. You can always ask someone for feedback to call attention to the areas you need to work on. Often we can't see our own faults until someone is willing to share them with us in a constructive way.

2. *Redefine* the way you approach relationships; it's an always evolving process. Try new styles and see how others respond and how you feel. Eventually you will find your way if you continue to pay attention and pat yourself on the back when you handle a tough situation correctly. Make a mental note of how well that worked in your favor, and try to recreate and use the technique again and again.

3. *Repeat* the process over and over to master it so it flows with your style.

4. *Relax* and focus on building an authentic positive connection. When you are coming from the heart, others will be more receptive.

What do you want people to feel and take away from your energetic exchange?

Focus on key messages and points you want to get across. Look for the audience's body cues and responses. Feel their energy and vibration to modify yourself, your behavior, and your content, including aspects like tone and body language.

### JOURNAL: Chapter 6

1. Write down what emotional intelligence means.
2. Write down things that may trigger an automatic reaction from you.
3. Write down ways you can control your reactions.
4. Write down activities that make you flow and glow.
5. Write down nonverbal cues you want to remember, and post them up wherever you do your video calls to remind yourself.

Gratitude Journal: Keep your gratitude attitude going with writing every day in your gratitude journal. It will help keep your cells thinking and feeling positivity!

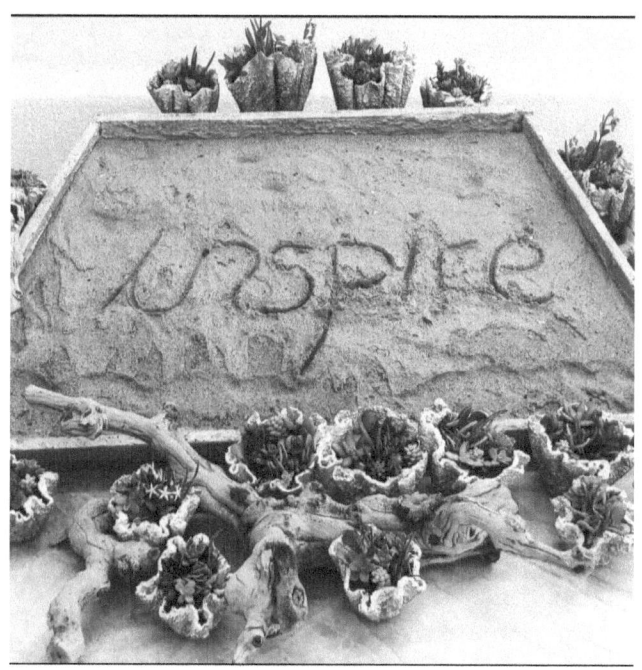

# CHAPTER SEVEN

# STRATEGIES

## STUDY STRATEGIES

If you ever struggle with a school subject, seek out a tutor. Everybody has different learning styles. Tutors can assess your situation and direct you to the best techniques to enhance your learning style. Once you know your learning style, a whole new world of possibilities opens up. Why? Because you can apply this knowledge in your life to accelerate and magnify your superpowers.

Let's cover the basics when it comes to learning styles; this way you can get an idea of what works best for you and begin to incorporate it immediately. The following is a breakdown of the different styles and percentages on how people learn. This is a key component to understanding the best strategies to use when it comes to mastering your mind and your overall life.

Here are retention rates for different forms of information processing, according to the National Training Laboratory's "learning pyramid":

- Lecture: 5 percent
- Reading: 10 percent
- Audiovisual: 20 percent
- Demonstration: 30 percent
- Discussion: 50 percent
- Doing: 75 percent
- Teaching others: 90 percent

Most people don't learn just from reading. I am a big fan of highlighting and going back to read the highlighted items. However, I know many students don't own the books, so I recommend using a pencil to underline important points. This way you can go back and reread the points over and over. When you are done, just erase all the marks you made, and the book is good as new.

I find I incorporate more than one style when it comes to learning. I read, I write, I listen, and I say it out loud. I'll be giving you a few tips in this chapter on how I imbed the information in my head, as well as more detailed descriptions of the different types of learning styles to review.

## Types of Learning Styles

1. Verbal: speaking information out loud, enabling the words to vibrate through the body. Write notes and highlight important points.
2. Aural: audible tones resonating information to the brain. Record to memory through hearing and listening.
3. Visual: using charts, colors, symbols, boxes, and emojis in note-taking.
4. Physical: utilizing the body and sense of touch to comprehend. Hands-on learning by moving, touching, building, and doing.
5. Social: learning through the collective group rather than swinging solo. Generate ideas through brainstorm sessions.
6. Logical: asking questions to get the whole picture. Categorize by thinking about patterns and in abstracts.
7. Solitary: preferring to spend time on their own. More introspective, independent, and intuitive.

## Chapter Books System

I want to share ideas on how to study smarter.

When I was younger, I was always looking for shortcuts and systems I could put into place when it came to processing information. I took a speed-reading class that was offered in high school. I don't know if they offer those classes anymore, but you can look up the technique on YouTube. In the class, we used our pointer finger and middle finger together to quickly scan the written lines on the page. Often I didn't feel like I was comprehending the information I was reading, but I practiced over and over.

I would use speed-reading from time to time but still didn't feel like I was maintaining the data. Often I found myself rereading a paragraph over and over, trying to retain the info. Then one day I decided to take a pencil to my book and start underlining the important information I knew a teacher might test on—dates, names, word definitions. I would then type up an outline of the chapter we were studying, and I would use that chapter outline as a study guide. I would read it several times a day. They say you tend to remember things when you read them first thing in the morning and right before you go to bed at night. So that is what I did.

Writing the outline stamps an imprint in your brain, kind of like a computer file. It also got my typing speed up rather quickly, which is a good thing because my brain still thinks faster than I can type. Reading the outline out loud is another way of learning. And come to think of it, you could record the outline in your voice on your phone and listen to it as you walk your dog or fold laundry.

As I've said, people learn in many different ways. And I found layering them worked best for me. I found reading, highlighting, typing an outline, and reading the outline several times throughout the day as well as in the morning and at night helped me score higher. Often I would continue to jam it into my mind right up to the point of taking the test. Then I would go back to the book and erase my pencil marks. Nobody taught me this technique. I just figured out a system that worked for me.

## Spelling Words System

When my daughter was in fifth grade, she needed to learn spelling words. I had found spelling to be very hard at that age and disliked it very much. Put me in front of a room in a spelling bee, and I thought I was gonna pee my pants. I did become runner-up in one spelling bee, but I believe it was sheer luck from the words I got.

My daughter was facing the same struggles. However, we developed a system—one that anyone can master.

Here is the system I came up with. Tests were on Fridays.

Monday

1. Write spelling words five times.
2. Quiz = written

Tuesday

1. Rewrite missed spelling words
2. Re-quiz = written
3. Verbally ask her to say the word, spell the word, and say the word again, just like in a spelling bee; she is now developing a mental photo.

Wednesday

1. Verbally quiz missed words like a spelling bee.
2. Quiz = written
3. Rewrite any missed words five times each.

Thursday

1. Quiz = written
2. Spelling bee, all words
3. Rewrite five times any misspelled words.

Friday

1. Rock the spelling test.

This system was successful for her. She felt good about herself when she noticed the results. In order to help her and myself remember the process, I printed the week out and taped it on the wall. Soon she was scoring higher than her friends whose parents were teachers. So that confirmed that what we were doing was working.

• • •

## SCHOOL SUBJECTS

### English

I went to a private all girls' Catholic high school taught by nuns in the '80s. Their goal was to make strong, smart women.

I had English right after lunch, and we had no air-conditioning in our classroom. Now, if you wonder what puberty, food, and heat does for a body, it leads to sleepiness. And I was not the only one; all the girls were sleepy. We were growing, the room was hot, and our bellies were full. We often found ourselves tuning out and dozing off.

My English teacher, Sister Anne, was quite the scary character. She was an older woman who walked with canes from having polio as a kid, and when she walked by one of our desks, she would smack her cane on the desktop, making us all jump in our seats. We never knew when it coming. She would always say, "Chew and digest." That was her slogan.

I wasn't a fan of English at that time. She forced us into an uncomfortable learning style for a class I disliked. No one wanted her as their English teacher. By the end of the semester, I was happy to get away from that scene. However, something must have stuck. I believe that writing has always been in my genes and I just didn't know it yet. Sister Anne was activating my superpowers, and I was resisting.

As I grew older, I worked with a book called *The Artist's Way* by Julia Cameron, which guides you to wake up and write several pages every morning. It's a popular book to this day, and I would recommend it to anyone who wants to get better at writing.

When I was older and my son was about seven years old, I reached out to my old high school to see if Sister Anne was still alive. I learned she was at a retirement nunnery and decided to take my son over to meet her. I wanted to thank her for teaching me to be the good writer I am today. I wanted her to know that she really made a difference in this world.

She was in a wheelchair and in a rundown environment by today's standards, but it was a beautiful exchange and a memory I am glad to have. I gave her the gift of appreciation, acceptance, and gratefulness, and imprinted a positive memory into her soul, as well as my own and my son's, while modeling the gift of acknowledgment. She died not long after, and I was grateful I had given my thanks for her service before she left this planet.

## Mathematics: Left Brain, Right Brain

I am left handed, which might have helped me in math. For some reason, I could do math in my head with half the steps. I didn't see a point in doing all that work the long way when I could cut it down and get the same answer. But for some reason the teachers only taught the long way.

Teachers would mark me off when I took a quiz or test because I didn't show my work. They thought I was cheating—until one day when the teacher asked one row of the class to go to the chalkboard to do a problem in front of the entire room. I don't know if teachers still do this today, but it can be intimidating, especially if you are struggling with a subject. We lined up, and the teacher gave us a long-division problem. I wrote the problem, cut the steps in half, and came up with the right answer in moments. I knew what I was doing, and the other girls always looked over to see if their answers matched mine. They knew I was good at math, but they couldn't copy because they didn't know how I was doing it.

It was at that moment that my teacher realized I was processing the information on a different level and that I could still gain the correct answer doing it my way. I share this with you to let you know there are multiple ways of doing things if given the right perspective. Math may be processed differently for you, depending on your mindset. When I look back now, I really believe math came easily to me because I can use both sides of my brain and access information most people cannot due to my being left handed. I believe the future of the new earth is using both sides of the brain to access more knowledge, problem-solving skills, coding, mathematical elements, and to detect the invisible.

When I tested for math in college, I tested for the highest level right out of the gates, which was finite business math. This meant I only had to take one math class, and then I was done with the subject in college forever. But I blew it. The class was Monday, Wednesday, and Friday at 8:30 a.m., and I was too busy partying and sneaking into bars to get up early to attend the class. When I tested again years later, I didn't test so high, and I had to start again at a lower level.

When you are on a roll and building momentum, that is the time to push yourself and not mess around.

## History

I love history for some reason. I liked learning about all the customs and faraway lands and events before our time. People were different back then. They didn't have it so easy. True trailblazers. Use the chapter books system to get through this class.

## Science

I was not a fan of science back in high school, but this attitude evolved as I grew older. Memories of looking through magnifying glasses, dissecting a pig, and learning about eye color and DNA sequences are what stick in my mind. A topic you may not like at a young age can change with perspective as you grow and learn. By far, science is one of the neatest topics when it comes to changing the world rapidly and magically. The chapter books system also works well here.

## Music

In fifth grade, I wanted to do something different when it came to playing an instrument. I wanted to play what a boy would play. My parents nixed the drums; I am sure they didn't want to live through me letting out my frustrations. So I chose the saxophone. It was edgy, different, and I was of course the only girl who played that instrument. Most of the girls chose violin, clarinet, or flute. However, I have to say it wasn't the best choice. I didn't think about the fact that I had to walk to and from school while carrying one of the heaviest instruments. I quickly ditched it.

In high school, I thought being in the band was for geeks. Now I realize musicians are some of the most enlightened people on the planet. They vibrate at higher frequencies and different levels, which allows them to access data not everyone can reach. My sister played the flute, and she went on to join the marching band in high school, while I did drill team. She played rather beautifully and fluidly.

Becoming a musician is not a guaranteed paycheck, so many families squash that option. However, I have met some amazing, talented musicians who never made it big. I would encourage every family to put your kids into some kind of music class at least once in their life. We all need exposure to really appreciate this art. Music is frequency used in the past, present, and future to heal humans on a cellular level, which makes it a very impactful, sought-after skill set. I urge you all to take a closer look at understanding frequency healing and trying new modalities in order to create your own self-healing strategy.

## STEAM: Science, Technology, Engineering, Art, and Math

New generations are so lucky to have these programs available. Combining and grouping these academic disciplines impacts workforce development, creating great leaders and entrepreneurs. Learning how to incorporate, intertwine, and integrate these subjects makes you very well rounded.

I've always said I am a Jill of all trades, meaning I've dabbled in many skills rather than gaining expertise by focusing on one. "Jack of all trades" is often a compliment for a person who is good at fixing and has a very broad knowledge. I became a Jill of all trades through my passion for learning, studying, growing, and evolving. I outgrew many people around me because I wanted to keep progressing and was always adding to my skill set. STEAM offers a more in-depth understanding of subjects and will help guide the planet to education, expansion, and evolution. Women are becoming leaders in technology and art, which was not the case in the past. STEAM is an access point for guiding students, dialogue, and critical-thinking skill sets.

• • •

## STEAMS/STEAMM: SCIENCE, TECHNOLOGY, ENGINEERING, ART, MATH, SOUND/MUSIC

Eventually I believe this will turn into STEAMS or STEAMM, the last *S* standing for sound or the *M* for music. Sound is the expression of universal mind source (universal language to all species), creating a one-mind synergy. Sound and music create vibratory paths to parallel dimensions that provide knowledge, wisdom, and the ability to astral project. Astral projection/astral travel is out-of-body travel when the soul separates from the body and your consciousness travels through the universe in order to access invisible information traveling in the air and through other dimensions. Sound is made up of particle waves that affect us. These particle waves can heal the body and send information to the mind and heart when ignited properly.

I believe I have gone into astral travel at times when writing this book, in order to get the messages I am supposed to share with you. In addition, I also do believe I have also achieved states of time or space travel in order to be able to see projections of the future as well as move into a technique called remote viewing. Remote viewing is a form of mental imagery where one can view a distant location, a person, event, or object. Basically, you can think about something and project your consciousness to move into that realm and take a look around the area to see what is taking place. There have been times when I have gone into remote viewing even when I didn't plan to, when the universe wanted to show me something it wanted me to see. When you work with energy and move through space, time, and the holographic field, you are working with multiple capabilities overlapping. I have been doing guided imagery since I was a kid, so this kind of technique came naturally to me without any proper training. I do believe that in the future, our children will be guided and trained to working with these amazing superpower modalities.

I work myself into that deep meditative state before I sit down to write by doing a combination of things.. I create an energetic platform where we are all united with our minds. I believe I am going into the eighth, ninth, tenth, eleventh, and twelfth chakras to access this information. I home in on you and receive ideas on what I need to share with you. This is unusual information in some cases.

## 5G Again

Today, I had no idea what area I was supposed to focus on until the messages come pouring in. I believed the book was almost completed, but I was directed to go back in and add this particular section. When I write, I put on calming yet elevating music that helps me transcend my mind to levels out of the norm as the music notes carry the vibrational frequency of information right into my third eye and above my head. I pull them in when I am relaxed and in the receiving mode of just letting go and letting it flow.

Remember how I told you there are vibrations, frequencies, and energies all around us that we cannot see or hear? Many people have been writing them off for years. Well, I am being told that inaudible sound frequencies all around us are affecting us mentally, emotionally, and physically. And I don't want to scare you, but it is directly related to 5G, radiation, electronic devices, satellites, phones, computers, microwaves, routers, etc.

I know a lot of you will want to read this book on an electronic device. And I am going to encourage you once again to work with hard copies if at all possible. The devices people use to read e-books are not good for the human body over long periods. Electronic data can also be easily modified, erased, or removed. A hard copy you can highlight, write in, bookmark, and use as a reference guide for life is the best kind.

What I have learned and recall from my memory database is that sound travels five times faster through water, and since our bodies are made up of close to 70 percent water, all those frequencies are traveling right through our bodies at very rapid speeds, whether the effect is positive or negative for us. We need to wake up and pay attention to this. I believe the power of sound is crucial for our new-earth movement toward conscious expansion, healing fragments of the soul. Sound will one day be the ultimate healing tool of humanity.

Our superpowers are being diminished in the name of faster Wi-Fi, better devices, and high technology. All this is hijacking our nervous systems, wreaking havoc, and messing up our human antenna; to decipher the codes, we need to be able to read the energies and frequencies clearly.

Many countries have been boycotting 5G over the years, but it has overtaken them as well. And certain countries push the 5G concept; I believe they do this in order to gain total worldwide power and control. I want you to be awake and aware so you can be empowered to make better choices for yourselves, your families, and your communities.

## Sound and the Pyramids

What I have learned about studying the pyramids and how they were built:

- Certain octaves and frequencies can turn solid objects to liquid. This technique was used to build the giant pyramids.
- Pyramids send electricity all over the earth.
- Pyramids charge the atmosphere, and the electricity charges the ground.
- Pyramids were built to be seen from above.
- A pyramid generates more energy than fifty nuclear power plants.
- Pyramids are generators of free positive energy and portals. They primarily function as stargates, which allow you to astral travel.
- Pyramids surpass human understanding.
- Pyramids affect and effect the psychic, mental, and astral energy of each person.
- Energy flow: Pyramid frequency is compatible constructive interference with the human aura and energy. Pyramid frequency is the opposite to Wi-Fi and invasive microwave electromagnetism.
- Pyramids bring a certain frequency to the planet and can immerse a human into higher vibrational frequencies.
- Pyramid frequency helps achieve things that aren't supposed to exist, such as levitation and moving objects mentally.

- Work through vibration synching, reflecting and vibrating at the same frequency as other pyramids
- Natural hub or amplifier for consciousness
- Compressed sound source
- Sonic levitation by sound

Sound and music align our superpowers, offering the power to create, liquify, energize, reach higher realities, achieve higher self, raise vibration, use mathematics, and receive much knowledge and extrasensory perception.

Remember, I am presenting information that may be new for you. Stay open, and you will expand with me.

I truly believe the power of sound and frequency have been way overlooked. Music class was part of the academic curriculum back in the 1980s and 1990s when I grew up and was eventually removed from the system. It is time to bring it back, front and center, so we can expand and learn more of these healing capabilities.

• • •

## BOOKS

Reading is a superpower. It expands your knowledge and imagination to allow for infinite creation. Have you noticed how difficult it can be to buy books these days? Everything has gone digital. What would happen if the internet were shut down? How would we learn? Would there be a panic or frenzy?

Owning a book allows you to bookmark it, write in it, and refer back to it. I went to Barnes and Noble to do some research and noticed their supply is limited; I could order online, but then I can't see the full content to judge whether the book will fulfill my needs. When I started writing this book, I wanted to go to a used bookstore to pick up some books to have on hand should the internet go down and I needed to teach my daughter. There are only two used bookstores around me, and they are in other cities, owned by only one culture. That was when it hit me. There was no place to go. We are forced to read digitally on our devices, which subjects us to their radiation twenty-four seven. Not the best idea.

So, once again, I am going to encourage hard copies of books. You know what else I know about books? The books on your shelf create a cloud of floating information around you that you can tap into anytime. I see this information as words of invisible light dancing in the air. You can access it when you tap into higher frequencies. You would be surprised how many times I have pulled a book I have read off the shelf to research a subject from years ago. Having access to good information right where you marked it is a powerful tool. Back in the day, libraries were respected, and many homes dedicated an entire room to literature. You were considered educated and wealthy when you had a library. When a culture wants to remove or change history, they burn books. Don't let history repeat.

Build a collection of books and use them to your advantage. I have a feeling that one day you will be very impressed with the knowledge you have acquired.

## DETENTION

My dad was an alcoholic who died of a heart attack at the young age of forty-three. I was seventeen and in my last year of high school. My mother and stepfather said if I wanted to graduate from Rosary High School, I had to pay my way through. I went after financial assistance, worked my tail off, and ponied up the cash.

We had moved to a new city a few years prior, and I had briefly attended a local high school where my race was a minority. I was treated poorly by the girls, and one day, I had about nine of them stalking me to kick my ass as I walked home from school. I approached the Spanish teacher in the classroom and said, "You see all those girls outside, looking in the window? They want to beat me up. Would you mind driving me home?" She agreed, and the girls followed us out to her car and watched me get in to drive away. I never returned.

So there I was at this pivotal crossroads, trying get over the loss of my father. Now, that was a big healing episode. I grew to imagine him as my guardian angel, always watching over me. It gave me strength to know I had him by my side. I would tell myself, *Nobody else has their dad by their side twenty-four seven like I do.* There have been times I've felt sad even as an adult, wondering what life would have been like if he had walked me down the wedding isle, what kind of advice he would have given me—on buying a car, navigating life, handling boys growing into men, children, and such.

I didn't have much family support in my teen years due to an unstable home environment. With two working parents and abusive stepparent issues, I often was given adult responsibilities. My mother had another child when I was seventeen, and I refused to have anything to do with him. I wasn't the one who got pregnant, requiring me to ruin my freedom to evolve. I didn't want yet another responsibility on my shoulders.

I worked until midnight many nights during the week at Medieval Times. Getting up to be at school at 8:05 a.m. was quite the challenge since I was tired and still growing. Often I would sleep in and go in late. The consequence was a forty-five-minute after-school detention—a small price to pay for a few more hours of sleep. At detention, we were instructed to write and copy some written content they gave us. As a left-handed person, I decided to make good use of my time and teach myself how to write with my right hand. Eventually I got really good at it. It was legible, so mission accomplished.

Taking a crappy situation and turning it into a positive is crucial to evolving. Kids sitting in detention are probably living miserable lives. I believe they are misunderstood, unacknowledged, dismissed, disrespected, abused, or may be invisible in their own minds. If this is you, I want to help equip you with the info you need to identify improper behaviors and work your way through the world as well as anyone else who listens in order to improve. The lessons of life often come when you are in the middle of a storm, during a deep transformation. It's uncomfortable as heck, but when you get out of the storm, you blossom like a flower because you were watered and doused with information and clarity. Healing my soul has always been my goal. I think when you heal the soul, you move up into other dimensions and realms to reach ascension when you leave this planet.

• • •

# CAREER DEVELOPMENT

## Young Career Development

When my son was about eight years old, I decided I wanted to expose him to professions he might be interested in pursuing when he got older. We didn't have the internet back then, so I reached out by phone to people we could interview to learn more about their jobs. I wanted him to ask about the best schools for their career, the costs, the typical workday, hours expected to work, and salary. We interviewed several types of architects, since he was an avid builder of Legos. I took notes, and we learned a lot about these professionals' experiences and what could be expected if he took that route.

Though encouraging your child's interests should start as soon as they're born, I highly recommend trying this particular method when your children are older than eight. My son still remembers it to this day and says he was too young at the time. But I tried. The memory is there, so it stuck. I am all about going straight to the right person to gain the knowledge needed to make magic happen.

## High School Career Development

When my son was in high school, I discovered he could take Cisco software college classes. Since his dad did information technology as a living, we were aware of this in-demand skill. So I signed him up and paid $400 for the class. It was after school at the Adult Learning Center not far from our house. We soon discovered that since he was in high school, the classes were free. Yes, you read that right. I am not sure if they still offer this incentive, but it would well be worth your while to check into it if you are interested.

At my son's age, I thought his father and I were going to have to deal with his getting drunk at parties, drugs, girls, and lots of poor learning choices. But my son chose to dive into the world of computers. At the time, I thought video game addictions were better than drug addictions, alcohol problems, crime, or teen pregnancy. But my son didn't want to apply himself in school. The addiction alarmed me. This didn't seem normal.

We finally took him to video game addiction counseling. Today I hear many parents talking about this concern, which is exactly why I bring up this point. Go back and reread the section on the digital matrix in this book, and you will see the patterns. Addiction to the internet, social media, and video games is claiming the souls of human beings. I can spot this because I have witnessed it over and over, disconnected myself, and controlled the mind manipulation.

Years later, I realized my son is a genius in his own way. He never applied himself in high school because he didn't like the environment, people, judgment, classification, etc. Let's face it: those are some of our most uncomfortable years. When kids are different, it is because they are operating at a unique frequency level and perspective. We need to get on their level and on all levels to elevate them to achieve their dreams. Many highly intelligent people are able to see, understand, and comprehend things most people don't notice or care to pay attention to, but being highly intelligent makes it hard to relate to others. This is not an easy road to travel.

You all have special abilities; maybe you just haven't been taught how to access your superpowers. By analyzing your kids' capabilities to their fullest extent, you can place them right where they need to be to thrive. Genes are an important factor.

So I tell you this: don't squash your kids, don't judge your kids, and don't label your kids. Encouragement over discouragement.

• • •

## FAMILY

Create a family if you feel you are not supported mentally, emotionally, or physically by your own blood. That is what counselors, therapists, coaches, doctors, mentors, healers, and friends are for. "Proud" was not part of my biological family's vocabulary. And as far as I am concerned, people can never hear "I am proud of you" and "I love you" too much in their lifetime. I adopted friends who became like sisters and older men who guided me and whom I called "Dad."

When my daughter gets out of the car at school, I make it a point to yell affirmations after her—things I want ringing in her head as she takes on the day: "You are a rock star"; "Go show the world who you are"; "Be magic"; "Be fabulous"; "You are beautiful"; "I love your hair"; "You are awesome"; "I am proud of you"; "I love you."

Create the life you want to have for yourself. You are the only person who can do it. You are here on this planet to be independent.

I half jokingly picked up this sign in a store and had my friend snap the photo. But in reality, this is how I've felt most of my life. Be your own cheerleader, and build your own cheerleading team.

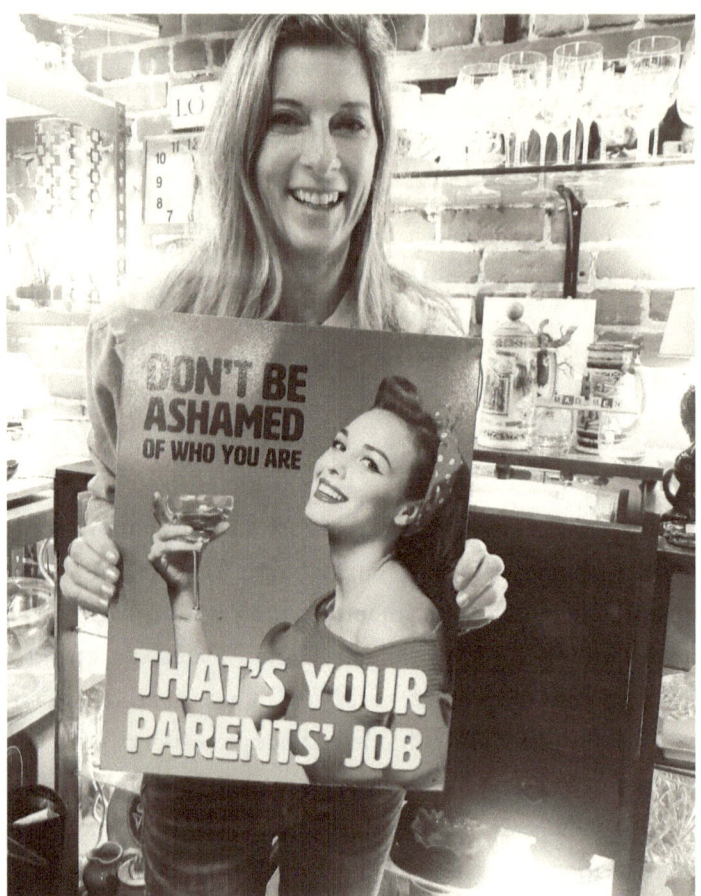

## CAREER DAY

Years after I graduated Rosary High School, alumni were invited to spend the day sharing information about our careers with the students. I've attended this event several times over the years. I felt I had a lot to give back, especially since a family had donated money for me to be able to finish my senior year with financial aid.

Typically the day would start out with a school assembly announcing the event and introducing us. Each of the girls was provided a list of the speakers' professions and got to pick which classrooms they would attend to learn about us and what we do. Each room's presentation usually consisted of three of us speaking for about ten minutes each. As time went on and I grew more experienced, I started typing out—you guessed it—an outline to hand out to the girls. I had so many life experiences I wanted to share to help the girls prepare for their futures.

One particular year, I typed up three pages. And lucky me: I was put in a classroom to speak alone for the entire thirty minutes because of a few no-shows. I still have the sheet, dated April 27, 2007, and I am going to include what it said when I wrote it at age thirty-six:

1. Let me say that your career search should not end here. I highly recommend each of you interview at least three different people in three different careers you are interested in pursuing. Ask them what their typical day is like, what you can expect on the job, the pros and cons of each position, and what type of salary one can expect. Often times we pursue something, but when we get into it, it is not what we expected.

2. Start saving for retirement from the moment you start working. People are living longer these days due to technology and medicine, and we haven't planned properly for it, let alone for the astronomical rising cost of healthcare, and it is only going to get more expensive in time. You can set aside 3 percent [I would say 10 percent in 2023] now and have your money working for you and up a steady retirement. Often people wait too long and then have to take out 12 percent [I would say 20 percent in 2023], which is a pretty big chunk to try and make up for the difference, because they don't have time on their side to build the fund. Build your fund now because one day, if you are lucky, you will make it to be a senior citizen, and don't you want to have a good retirement lifestyle?

3. Learn to be good with money, budget, and live within your means. Don't get a bunch of credit cards and go crazy. Credit card companies target students, especially college kids who are just getting into the credit system. You are the next generation

they are trying to hit to make their interest money off. If you charged $100 and didn't pay it off and it has a 26 percent interest rate, you now owe $126. That is more than 25 percent or one-fourth of the money used. You are held responsible for paying off the credit you acquire even if you don't have a job.

We are now in the day and age where we have to watch our credit because of scam artists. Make sure you shred anything with personal information before placing it in the trash. This is how identity theft starts, so don't make it easy, and protect yourself. I do a personal credit check every year just to make sure the credit accounts I have open in my name correspond. You will also be graded on how often you pay your bills on time, how much you pay off vs. how much debt you acquire. This is called a FICO score. Your FICO score is pulled up anytime you want to make a big purchase, such as a home or a car. You will get a better interest rate on the money you borrow if you have a high score. The goal here is to live within your means.

4. Another money issue that nobody ever told me but has worked out to my advantage is to keep a separate banking account from your spouse or boyfriend. Often women give this up when they get married or have children. It is important not to give your mate all the control. You need to be aware where the money is going and how it is being distributed and be part of the budget. More often than not, women give up control, and if their spouse dies or leaves them, they have no idea how to deal with the finances and are often left in debt and don't have a clue as to how to distribute life's expenses, nor do they know how much money they will need per month to survive comfortably.

5. Have a will and trust. It is important when you buy your home to put it in a trust; otherwise, if your property goes to probate,

the state can take up to 10 percent of its value. By having it in a trust, you eliminate the state's cut, and the money will go to whomever you have placed in charge of the trust. You will acquire items of value throughout the years. It may be a home, a business, a boat, a motor home, your savings accounts, etc. In order to protect them, you are also going to want a will stating who your belongings are to go to.

You may also find yourself being faced with something called a power of attorney when you go to the doctor's office. It is a signed statement that if you are in a situation where you are not capable of making healthcare decisions for yourself, such as being in a coma, a spouse or a family member will be in charge of the decision-making process. Often it is best to discuss with whomever you put in charge how you would like the issue handled. [In 2023 I say call a family meeting to go over your wills and trusts by telling everyone who gets what and how it will be handled. That way it comes directly from your mouth and you can let it be known to all in one shot. Shoot video of the family meeting, and put it with your documents to be viewed after you pass. That way you have complete confirmation of your wishes, and no one can try to override anyone else.]

6. It is important to present yourself in the correct manner. When it comes to dressing professionally for your job, hot and hip is not in the job description. Save the low-cut tops and crop tops for the clubs. Women will hate you, and men will not respect you. Accessorizing goes a long way. Pump it up with fun jewelry, tactful hair and makeup, killer shoes, and happy handbags.

7. Gossiping in the workforce will come back to bite you in the butt. It is better not to say anything at all if you can't say something nice. I know you have been hearing this since you

were a kid, but it holds true. Cussing is also something you do not want to do. It represents not having any class and being uneducated.

8. You have the capability to learn anything you want to. Knowledge is power. In order to progress in life, you need to constantly evolve, so learning never ceases. If you want to know how to do something, get up and go learn about it and do it. Read books, use the web. You are the smart women of the world. History is in the making; women are finally being seen as equal in the workforce.

9. Anybody ever watch the show *Apprentice*? You can learn so much from watching how the interviewees handle the long, drawn-out job interview. Observe how they cope with job pressure, their organizational skills, how they speak and act. Learn to duplicate the traits you see as an asset. It can be as simple as holding your body posture, learning how to present yourself or how to shake hands. Have a firm handshake; it shows confidence. . . .

10. Bearing children changes your body, and they change you mentally, emotionally, and physically. If you have a child, you are going to be faced with "Do I work or stay home?" It is all about trying to find the right balance for you and your family and what kind of lifestyle you choose to lead.

11. Remember what I said about separate bank accounts? You need to split up the household chores with your spouse/mate right from the get-go. Otherwise you could be accountable for much more than the man on the home front.

12. Each one of us is on our way to becoming a senior citizen someday. More and more I am seeing the need for adult day-care centers, assisted-living communities, hospice care, etc. As people age, they can't take care of themselves, have limited mobility or disabilities, and need other people's help to survive.

I have brought information books that are geared toward guiding seniors to find the services they need. Help yourself to them if you are interested in getting an idea of their needs, services, or jobs.

13. Go to college, and go after any college scholarships you can, even if your parents can afford it, because it is pricey. Take out a loan if you have to. Get the whole college experience. You only get one chance to do it right. Yes, you can go when you are older, but it is not the same. You will get paid more for the rest of your life because you have a college degree. Nice guarantee.

14. Alcohol will impair your judgment, so be extra cautious about what you are saying, doing, and the signals you are giving. Do not get intoxicated at work functions or holiday parties; it ruins your reputation and credibility instantly. You may be in situations with men that are uncomfortable, awkward, or unusual. Some men prey upon women, so protect yourself and listen to your sixth sense. It may take some time to develop your sixth sense and hear it, but it develops as you age, and with experience comes good judgment.

15. Wear sunglasses to protect your eyes, which in turn prevents you from squinting. This will help with crow's feet and wrinkles around the eyes, as well as protect your vision. Wear sunscreen, and use the self-tanner lotions to prevent from getting skin cancer and wrinkles. [In 2023 I would say no to self-tanners; they are full of toxic chemicals, and natural skin color is "in."]

16. And the last great tidbit I'd like to share with you is to make a list of the things you would like to do in your twenties, thirties, and forties, or maybe by the time you are a certain age. Set some goals and have fun; it could be to go to a nude beach, meet a famous person, and travel to Spain. Aim to accomplish the things you would like to do in your lifetime, and be willing

to change them as you grow—because your ideas will change, and so will you, through knowledge, education, and the wisdom of experience. It feels great to see goals written down and checked off so you can look back on your life and see all your accomplishments. It will remind you of who you are, how far you have come, and what helped shape you into the woman you want to be.

17. In closing, you are going to be faced with a lot of choices in your lifetime. You are in charge of your own destiny, so it is up to you to make the best choices for yourself. I hope I have shared something with you that will make a difference in your life, now and forever.

    Thank you for having me.

It's been years since I did that presentation, and I have evolved, so the content in this book has also evolved. The teacher sitting in the back of the room was mesmerized by the vast amount of information pouring out of my soul so passionately in such a short period of time. I knew I only had thirty minutes to fit in a lifetime of lessons.

I looked forward to these special days. If I said just one thing that gave my audience that aha moment, mission accomplished!

## TRAVELING ABROAD

Regarding higher learning, I think more and more people will be opting for home study or may have no choice in the matter with the way the world is going—and that is unfortunate. In the past, traveling abroad was embraced, giving students more freedom. Traveling expands you and exposes you to life experiences filled with lessons on other cultures and people. Going to another country to get educated may be exactly what you need to do—especially if the school is well known for a certain subject.

People in other countries often speak three to four languages. Most Americans only speak one. We should change that.

## STAND UP

I find one of the best ways to tap into my creativity is to use a stand-up desk. When you stand up, energy flows through you differently.

Whenever I want to get really creative, I raise my desk and crank up happy music. Sometimes I step back and dance in between working and thinking so I can access more information to bring in. I recommend using a stand-up desk when it comes to anything you want to conquer. It's good for your back, your body, your posture, energy, and blood flow. I also like using it when I do video calls and meetings. It puts me more in my power of owning who I am.

## SUPERPOWER STANCE

One day when I got out of the shower, I stood there butt naked and separated my feet, put my hands on my hips, and announced to the world, "I am one of the strongest women on the planet." *I loved it.* Here I was at this moment of vulnerability, completely owning my own energy and life force. I realized I have been through a heck of a lot and became very proud of myself. The storms that I have faced, conquered, respected, and learned from made me realize I am pretty dang incredible. I recommend finding your own superpower stance, taking the position, and yelling out what you are to the world. You are claiming it, imbedding it in your body, and projecting it. Now, that is working your superpowers. No one can take this away from you.

· · ·

## FICO SCORE/CHECKBOOK/PAYING BILLS

What is a FICO score?

A FICO score is a three-digit number, typically on a 300-to-850 range, that tells lenders how likely a consumer is to repay borrowed money based on their credit history.

When I went back to college with kids half my age in 2014, I received a ton of credit card offers in the mail. That's when it hit me. We must prepare kids to look out for this, as I mentioned in my career-day presentation. When you enter college, you become part of the next generation of money borrowers that credit companies will target. Not paying off your credit card bill every month leads you to acquire something called interest. If you charged $1,500 and didn't pay it off and your interest rate is 20 percent, you now owe $1,800—$300 *more*. Isn't that insane? Then it continues to get added onto, month after month, if you don't pay it off. And you could have used all that interest money on things you really need.

Only get a credit card and use it if you plan to pay it off every month. This helps build your credit score to get the highest ranking. You will want a score 750 or above. Anyone over 800 can pretty much buy anything they want. But do they buy anything they want? No. That is why they have an 800-plus score. Make a list of the items you really need and stick to it. Set aside money for retirement and rainy days, when you really need it. Control yourself and purchases.

Being a minimalist is very much in. As you age, you acquire a house full of crap you don't want or need, and then you or your family has to figure out what to do with it. I have been in my house twenty-six years, and in 2022, I made five donation trips to Goodwill, and I can still clear more out my closet. I have worked with many seniors who are hoarders, and the amount of clutter they have collected can affect their health.

Having very little gives you the freedom to move around in the world without having to worry about junk in a storage unit. Most likely you will never get back to that junk, and someone will claim your unit and auction it off.

## Paying Bills System

Let me give you a strategy for paying bills. Gather your bills and a blank sheet of lined paper. I like to write mine out like this:

2022 Feb Bills Paid March:

| Living Expenses: | |
|---|---:|
| Mortgage/Rent | $3,300 |
| Water | $88.96 |
| Phone | $96.48 |
| Gas | $66.72 |
| Electric | $75.45 |
| Total | $3,627.61: cost per month to live in a dwelling |

| Credit Card Expenses: | |
|---|---:|
| Care Credit | $400.00 |
| Visa 1 | $1,545.26 |
| Biz Visa | $780.00 |
| Total | $2,725.26: |

cost of food, gas, car insurance, living expenses

Gardener Check #201 $50.00

Make sure you deduct these amounts from your checking account and balance out your account. It should look like this:

| Check# | Date | Transaction | Payment | ✓ | Deposit | ✓ | Balance |
|---|---|---|---|---|---|---|---|
| | | | | | | | **11,560.33** |
| | 2/24/22 | Marshall Mortgage | 3,300 | ✓ | | | 8,260.33 |
| | 2/24/22 | Water | 88.96 | ✓ | | | 8,171.37 |
| | 2/26/22 | Phone | 96.48 | ✓ | | | 8,074.89 |
| | 2/28/22 | Gas | 66.62 | ✓ | | | 8,008.27 |
| | 2/28/22 | Electric | 75.45 | ✓ | | | 7,932.82 |
| | 2/25/22 | Care Credit | 400.00 | ✓ | | | 7,532.82 |
| | 2/25/22 | Capitol One Visa | 1,545.26 | ✓ | | | 5,987.56 |
| | 2/25/22 | Chase Visa | 780.00 | ✓ | | | 5,207.56 |
| 201 | 2/25/22 | Gardener | 50.00 | ✓ | | | 5,157.56 |
| | 3/1/22 | PAYDAY | | | 15,000 | ✓ | **20,157.56** |

Your leftover balance in your account after paying bills is the bold number in the bottom right corner, and the one below it is your balance after a deposit has been made. Payment is subtracted from the total, which is then placed in the far-right balance column. Notice the second to the last row. The gardener was paid by check. Check #201 is listed in the left corner so you know what check number it is. Attached is how you write out a check. I will include some blank ones at the end of this chapter so you can practice writing a check.

Make sure you double-check your credit card statements to make sure you really did make those purchases and transactions. You need to track and monitor this to avoid improper use of your cards. Use the check marks in the smaller columns to note when the payment clears so you know the bill has been paid. Usually you do this when you go back the next month and pay your bills again.

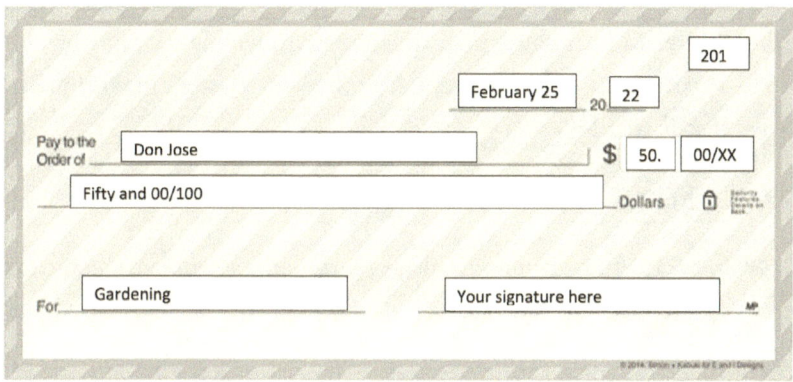

## Credit Cards

Let's talk more about credit cards here for a minute. As you can see from my paying bills example, I have a CareCredit card. I acquired this card because I had to have about $10,000 of dental work done. Dental insurance isn't like health insurance. It usually doesn't cover much, so you are stuck paying out of pocket. And the older you get, the more dental issues you will have. That is why it's important that you start saving at a young age.

The CareCredit card has zero interest if you pay if off within a certain amount of months. I make a higher payment than they are asking so I can pay it off before that time frame hits. Otherwise I will be paying 26 percent on $10,000, which is $2,600 for a total of $12,600. This credit card can also be used for cosmetic procedures. But remember: you need to pay it off prior to the deadline to reap the benefits.

Call your credit card companies to stay on top of the dates, or write them on a calendar. You will need to keep track. They will not remind you. Remember, this is how they make their money.

I recommend going online and doing the research for yourself when acquiring a credit card. Sure, you will get credit card offers in the mail if your credit is good. But chances are you can find a better deal if you shop them yourself. Many offer double points or other incentives such as zero interest for twelve months. If you maintain good credit, pay on time, and pay more than the minimum payment or pay off the balance, you are a credit card genius working the system in your favor. Now, that is strategy.

## AAA Card: $50 a year

When you start driving a car, I recommend getting an AAA card every year. Especially if you are a girl. If you get a flat tire, have a dead car battery, lock your keys in your car, or need your car towed, you can make a call, and someone will come and take care of you. It serves its purpose well when you need it and is a small price to pay when you are in this situation. The card also offers you hotel discounts, travel services, and other benefits.

• • •

# LIFE INSURANCE

If you own anything of value, have a life insurance policy. Life insurance pays out money to your kids and family when you die. Aim to have a decent amount that could pay off part of the house or leave your family without debt and with something to lean on. Let's face it: we are all going to die. No one wants to talk about it. But I do. It's a given fact, so prepare accordingly.

Term life insurance covers you for a specific amount of time. If you get a twenty-year policy, you're covered for that twenty-year term. That's it. So if you die after that twenty-year policy runs out, your family gets paid nada. Of course, this coverage is the cheapest and is mostly used when you have young kids.

Whole life insurance is a type of coverage that lasts your whole life. Whole life plans are more expensive than term insurance, but with good reason. Whole life insurance is designed to build cash value, which means it doubles as an investment account.

## WILLS, TRUSTS, POWER OF ATTORNEY, BINDERS

Since I worked with senior citizens for many years, I saw the writing on the wall. We are all going to get older—if we are lucky to make it that far—and pass away someday. I have witnessed the aging process and seen people who were and weren't prepared. Let me share ideas with you to help you prepare a bit and understand the process. No one teaches how to prepare for the aging process, so this should give you some insights.

- Wills: According to Wikipedia, wills are legal documents that express "a person's . . . wishes as to how their property . . . is to be distributed after their death and . . . which person . . . is to manage the property until its final distribution."
- Trusts: According to Investopedia, "Trusts are established to provide legal protection for the trustor's assets, to make sure those assets are distributed according to the wishes of the trustor, and to save time, reduce paperwork, and, in some cases, avoid or reduce inheritance or estate taxes."

Also from Investopedia:

> Unlike wills, which take effect upon death, trusts become effective upon the transfer of assets to them. . . . Trusts are frequently used in estate planning to benefit and provide for the distribution of assets to the heirs of the grantor. . . . In addition, trusts can be created to serve a variety of purposes,

both before and after the death of the grantor. During their lifetimes, grantors can create revocable trusts, which they can alter, amend, or terminate at any time. [The trust serves when someone becomes disabled.]

All I can say here is that when you own property, get a will or trust. You will save a ton of time, money, and energy for your family. Work with a trusted advisor and look it over from time to time over the years to make sure you still agree with its terms, or alter it if you want to make changes.

- Power of Attorney: A power of attorney is a written authorization to represent or act on another's behalf in private affairs, business, or some other legal matter, such as matters of health. Power of attorney grants to holder authority to act as the principal, grantor, or donor. When you get to a certain age, your doctor's office has you fill out this form. They want to know what to do with you if something drastic should happen. God forbid.

- Healthcare Binder: Do your research. That is what the internet is for. Keep a three-ring binder with printouts for each family member, compiling bloodwork, doctor visits, diagnoses, etc. You need to be in control of your health, and creating a personal healthcare manual is important. That way, when you switch doctors, you have it all in one place. You will switch doctors many times in your lifetime as insurance and jobs change. Take notes on which medications don't agree with you and which do. Or bodies change all the time, and so do the results.

    Traditional medicine and holistic health should go hand in hand. When I was younger, I just trusted that doctors would give me the right information. However, I have learned doctors are limited in their knowledge. They only know what they were taught and what they have witnessed. There are many advanced developments from other countries and natural approaches that work just as well, if not better.

When my son was seventeen and I took him to the doctor's office for an appointment, I asked him to fill out his intake forms. I wanted to go over them with him and help him prepare for this stage in his life. My mother never sat down to talk about these kinds of obligations with me, and I thought it was important to prepare my son for his own healthcare journey. Make creating a healthcare binder for each family member a priority; this way you can build a healthcare record they can take with them when they move out of the house, and all their records are in one place.

- Home Binder: Create a three-ring home binder for your house. This is a great place to put your home or renter's insurance policy (similar to a car insurance policy, only for a house), home receipts, and instruction manuals for appliances and other big purchases you make.

- Tax Files: Every year, you are going to have to file taxes. You will need to keep receipts of the items you purchase and hold onto them in case you get audited, which means the IRS comes knocking at your door to make sure you claimed the correct items. My advice here is to work with a professional tax preparer who knows the ins and outs and laws. You don't want to have to go through the stress of this all by yourself, and if you know you did everything by the book to the best of your abilities, you will be all right. I have a drawer dedicated to the receipts I collect throughout the year. At the end of the year, I separate them, enter them into an Excel spreadsheet, and bring the sheet to the tax guy with my needed forms to file. If you run your own business, it is best to have a separate credit card for that business. That way you can easily identify what was bought and spent by the business.

## Funeral

At the age of thirty-seven, I marched into a funeral home and said, "I want to plan my funeral." Shocked at my determination to talk about something so dark at a young age, the clerk directed me to the owner, whom I happened to know from networking in the senior industry. I was happy to have someone I knew to handle issues of such a delicate nature. We sat and discussed options: cremation versus burial, urns, costs, procedures, etc. He wanted me to put down a hefty deposit of thousands of dollars, claiming the price would only go up by the time I die. I said, "That is okay. I want to be cremated. That is the cheapest. Put it in my file. I have life insurance to cover that."

I literally sat down, wrote my desires on paper, and planned out my funeral. I wanted everyone to wear white clothing instead of black. None of this traditional crap for me. To me, white represents purity, angels, happiness, love, kindness, light, heaven. I wanted party balloons, Mexican food (an old family tradition), '80s music, a slideshow of fun photos streaming on the TV in the background, and I wanted butterflies released. And my ultimate favorite: a park bench in my city with my name on it, overlooking the park or the beach. I also wanted artists who felt compelled to connect with me to be able to come and paint my bench, making it stand out from the rest, just like I do. I asked the owner to file away my wishes until the time came.

In 2023, I still have the same requests, except I'd opt for a variety of music besides just '80s. I can't help it. I love all kinds of music.

• • •

## SCAM ARTISTS

There are several way to pay bills. Most people make payments online through their bank account. Protect this information! Never pay bills using a laptop on public Wi-Fi. This gives anyone and everyone access to your private login info, your bank, your account number, etc. No way José. Pay from a wired desktop computer if you can, in a private search window. Our present and future is riddled with thieves trying to steal our information and scam artists who want to take us down.

One day I received a call from a man who claimed he was going to arrest me because I didn't show up for jury duty. I find that these calls come when you are frazzled and least expect them; it's almost like they got your name off a list of people going through trauma. I was going through a divorce and getting ready to attend the Newport Beach Film Festival opening night to do their press/media, so I was pretty distracted. The guy kept me on the phone for forty-five minutes, threatening me and working me up—demanding that I pay him $2,500 or he was going to come to my house and arrest me in front of my kids.

I explained my situation, telling him I didn't even know I had jury duty and that I am a single mom, so I couldn't come serve anyway since I had to work to take care of my kids. He didn't care. He kept insisting I didn't serve my duty and I was going to pay a fine, or he was coming to arrest me. I was pissed that he thought it was okay to arrest me in front of my children. I drew the line.

I said, "Fine, since you say you are an authority and I have not met my duty, meet me down at the Huntington Beach Police Station, and I will work out the details with you there." *CLICK.* He ended the call. He was a total scam artist who stressed me out and wasted my precious energy and time. Never mess with a mother when it comes to affecting her children. We become lionesses and will turn the tables. Later I realized I had given him way too much personal information while defending myself. Be very careful of these scams.

## IRS Scam

I had a friend from junior high who was going through a divorce and got a call that she owed the IRS money and that she needed to pay immediately or she would be arrested. She was working multiple jobs as a single, full-time mother of two, struggling to make ends meet. When this call came in, her reaction was to put out yet another fire.

This scam artist filled her with so much fear that she drained her savings account of over $20,000 and turned it over to him, leaving her with nothing for her and her children. It all happened very quickly. He convinced her to drive to the bank and make a transfer. He wouldn't let her get off the phone to call anyone the entire time she was driving.

Pay attention to what is going on around you, to you, and with you. These scam artists prey upon people, looking for an opportunity to mess with you mentally to get what they want. Our minds are very powerful and can be triggered in an instant if caught off guard. She and her son ended up having to move in with me for a few months so I could help her get back on her feet.

## Multi-Level Marketing

Believe it or not, there are many companies out there preying upon women who are looking to better themselves and become independent. Many of these scammers promise big rewards, prizes ,and high commissions to top-producing product representatives. They display other women making it big, living the life, and having it all.

These companies often turn out to be pyramid schemes, where the ultimate goal is to get you under them, working your rear off, so they can receive commissions of your sales. They want you to sell to your family and friends and recruit, often not even supporting you in the process. I have to say, I have fallen victim to some of these pyramid schemes in my lifetime. Think twice before you jump into an independent sales role; research the product, talk to others about their interest in the products, and interview other consultants to paint a true picture of the outcome. Just know that everything you are generating is going right back to the top tiers; unless you are sitting on the very top, you are just a product peddler or a guinea pig purchasing their merchandise.

## Senior Citizen Scams

I have heard many horror stories of senior citizens being drained of their entire life savings and retirement. This is especially easy to do if they have memory problems. One time, I worked with a man who thought he had millions of dollars in the bank, and we wrote an offer on a property for $2.5 million. I went to the bank with him to get proof of funds, and the bank teller looked at me with sheer terror when she found that he didn't have any money in his bank account to live off of. At that moment, we realized he had been scammed and called in Social Security and Social Services to investigate.

Life can change in an instant.

## Cybersecurity

According to Wikipedia, "cybersecurity or information technology security is the protection of computer systems and networks from . . . information disclosure, theft of or damage to hardware, software, or [electronic] data, as well as from the disruption or misdirection of the services they provide." Thieves can steal private data and lock out the owners, thereby preventing their company from running so the attackers can demand a very high ransom fee. I have heard of cases where they demand four million on the first day, and then it goes up one million every day after. The company doesn't want to pay, thinking their IT department can fix it, but when they can't, they might end up paying seven million. It is a very real thing. There are high-paying jobs in information technology to secure networks from attacks.

If you are smart and want to protect yourself, do not create social media profiles. People who have ceased to exist online are the least tampered with because they have not shared their personal information. Protect yourself and data as much as you can by staying offline and off the grid.

• • •

## FOLLOWING GOOD LEADERS

I am all about working with coaches, therapists, mentors, healers, and counselors. But an important factor to consider is to only work with ones you trust. We all need good guidance in our lifetime. We are going to be faced with issues we have never faced before. Listen to your gut and pay attention to the vibrational details someone is giving off. Be careful of falling victim to illusion. Remember, we aren't limited to local support. We can go global thanks to the internet, Zoom, and social media. But with the digital matrix and the ability to access everyone worldwide, many celebrities are going online to try and drum up business using their fame to influence your decisions. I know you have noticed it with all the celebrity and influencer endorsements. A new platform on the rise, called Kyra, is grooming influencers to target and peddle products for placement and performance.

Others are creating grandiose coaching platforms, trying to influence humanity on a global level. How do I know this? In 2022, I took seven online coaching seminars and noticed the possible worldwide abuse of power taking place, which alarmed me very much. Many of these platforms offered personal coaching for upward of $20,000 per year, $7,000 per month for the top tier, with a $2,000 cancellation fee should you choose to opt out. Now, this isn't for the everyday people. These annual fees can equal someone's yearly salary in some cases. So, while I encourage coaching and working with people of knowledge, you must use your good judgment: ask yourself if you can afford it and if their values align with yours, and really pay attention to what they offer. If you can get a free ticket, I say take it and do it. That is what I did to level up: learn and discern.

Eventually, if a coaching program has people of high society involved as well as the average people from all over the world, they could take over the entire planet by domination and influence. We do not want one person running the entire planet. This will ruin us. When you hear Elon Musk talking about having to go to Mars, this is likely what he means. If we let AI or some entity overtake humanity, we will have to evacuate Earth to escape. Then again, I also believe there are already other species on Mars, so Elon might just be warming you up to the idea of what lies ahead in the future. As a futuristic visionary myself, I get hits of what is yet to come, which is why I composed this book—to help humanity envision what I see and alter their course accordingly.

I have followed people I thought were good leaders, only to discover that behind the scenes, they had ulterior motives: the desire to overtake the weak, conquer others, or act unethically and morally wrong in the name of financial gains, success, ego, and youth. They may look a certain way and preach that one thing you are all about, but in the end what they really want is to own your soul and life force for eternity. Be careful of falling victim to illusion.

## LINKEDIN

One place you might consider focusing your social media attention is LinkedIn. We all need to utilize this platform. I have learned from my coaches that LinkedIn is a very powerful platform when it comes to finding work, building a reputation, and making connections with influential people who have shared interests.

Did you know that for a small monthly fee, you have access to all sorts of classes—business development, Adobe Suite, marketing, etc.—that you can receive certifications for? And the certification attaches to your LinkedIn profile. Plus, you can print them out or save them on your computer. I took thirty-three LinkedIn learning classes during the pandemic and read nine books. I dove into learning and working on myself. I wasn't really fazed by the pandemic since I went within and didn't listen to media or watch news reports.

When I took a class, I would reach out to the instructor and thank them for their knowledge, asking for a connection. I even had one instructor, Dean Karrel, send me his book, called *Mastering the Basics*, simple lessons for achieving success in business. This book helped propel me into an industry I had never worked in before and a new career writing business proposals for a living. Future employers will be checking your LinkedIn profile; it is your online résumé. That is the one platform you want to show off your amazing skill sets and superpowers.

In high school, I was known by my friends as the writer. If we got into a fight, I would write a letter explaining my perspective, and once they understood it, we made up rather quickly. However, my mother never saw my writing capabilities. She always pushed me to get a job working for someone else. That was how she grew up. So I did what she made me feel I had to do—work for others who didn't respect, appreciate, or honor me for my talents and skill sets that I worked so hard to develop and grow.

At the age of fifty-one, I decided no more. I was going to have faith in me even if she didn't, and I told her that. Faith over fear. I made the jump. No regrets; an internal knowing kicked in: *I am going to follow my life purpose at all costs.* They say you really mature and get to the point where you don't care what others think at age fifty. I have arrived.

One of the purposes of this book is to help equip you with the tools to figure out your soul purpose before the age of fifty and follow it relentlessly. Don't let others dictate who you are. You decide. You will reinvent yourself multiple times in your lifetime. Have at it.

Something else I want to share here about LinkedIn is that when I am watching a documentary on TV or come across people doing neat things I want to learn about or be associated with, I reach out to them on LinkedIn by sending a message about how I enjoyed their project and requesting a connection. I give you this tip as a great way to get in touch with those you dream of working with, now or in the future.

Please feel free to connect to me on LinkedIn. I would love to hear your thoughts on this book. I am under Noelle Hipke (Hipkey TV).

## VOLUNTEERING: NEWPORT BEACH FILM FESTIVAL

Volunteer in your community for projects you are passionate about. It will well be worth your time and effort for the positive energy exchange. In 2010, I started volunteering for the Newport Beach Film Festival, doing their photography. It granted me the opportunity to meet filmmakers from around the world, learn cutting-edge techniques to help me evolve my skills, and get in contact with inspirational leaders.

As a Realtor, I wanted to be exceptional at worldwide storytelling. The Newport Beach Film Festival ignited me to go back to college and produce and direct a web series on the festival in 2014. (You can find it on YouTube under Hipkey TV.) Having zero experience, I threw myself on the red carpet and interviewed celebrities. I got Ted Baker to sponsor our clothing and eventually became a common face in the crowd, year after year.

I would take off work and dive into the event for the entire week, watching films and meeting the actors and filmmakers while interviewing whomever would answer my burning questions. I was intrigued with the costs, what cameras they used, how they did the lighting, how long the film took to shoot, where it was located, and other concepts. We'd all spend the entire week together, watching films, hanging at the after-parties, and meeting for seminars to hear speakers. Every year had a different vibe and unique energy. I always grew emotional at the end of the week; I never took for granted these once-in-a-lifetime events. I knew what we had just experienced was an energy exchange the likes of which would never happen again.

I most likely won't see many of these creators face-to-face again since they were from other parts of the world. The biggest takeaway for me was the creativity that flowed between us. My creativity levels tended to peak during those weeks I hung out with other creatives.

So, dive into what you are passionate about by giving back to others, and the rest will follow.

## INTERNET VERSUS LIBRARY

The internet is a library for researching and learning. Man, you guys have the universe at your fingertips, but a lot of negative baggage comes with it.

I used to hang out at the local library a lot because it was quiet and I could hear myself think. The local library is one of the healthiest places on earth to conduct schoolwork or study any area you want to focus on. Besides, the libraries have all the old books on hand that you can check out, make copies of, and use to your advantage. I highly recommend hitting up libraries in your area and the surrounding cities to dive into academics. Forget Starbucks or busy cafés; those are too noisy and aggravating to truly allow productivity. I think it's good to note here that librarians make decent money; this career may be worth looking into if you are a bookworm.

## SOCIAL MEDIA

I have got to write about this topic again. Social media sucks. I've been doing social media and videos since 2008. I spent much of my time living behind my phone and not in the present moment. I spent hours editing, creating, posting, liking, and waiting for others to like my posts. What I have learned is that social media is a toxic platform when it comes to your mind. Never have I experienced such deep emotions of not being good enough, envy for what other people are doing or have, jealousy that I wasn't included in a friend's event, and the list goes on. Friends would call crying about how it made them feel when they saw something that triggered them. So I stopped looking, stopped posting, and stopped interacting, and I am so dang happy.

Still, I have been doing social media for the Newport Beach Film Festival since 2010. Ironically, an entire Brazilian film was devoted to a girl who was struggling so badly with social media that she ended up committing suicide. And this cyberbullying is happening everywhere. Boys and girls, if you don't have anything nice to say, just don't say anything. Future employers are watching. Being online builds your reputation, good or bad, and the government is monitoring you. Your safest bet is to not engage or exist. Do not give anyone your personal info: what you like to do, where you hang out, who you are with, etc. You know what I am talking about here. You are beautiful people; you don't need to broadcast it. And if you are out of town and you feel that you must post pictures, do not post them until you return.

I have to admit, every once in a while, I will get back on social media to reach out to someone. I now follow inspirational quote accounts, positive influencers, and the like, and I only do it in very small doses—as in once every few days, for only a few minutes. I am sure I will have to launch back into it when I drop this book, but I will be doing so for the benefit of mankind.

## KILL THE DEVICES

In order for me to live my life seamlessly, my phone is pretty much always on silent mode during the day unless I am expecting a connection to come through. This way I am able to write without annoying distractions. Otherwise, useless information comes flooding in multiple times a day, trying to get me to buy this, read that, believe this, or go do that. My phone is trying to control, manipulate, and interrupt me. I refuse to give it power anymore. I drive off without it on purpose, knowing I am free from its chains. No one can track me, and I can soar as high as I want to go.

Turn off your devices at night—the Wi-Fi router, tablets, computers, phones, etc.—and use a regular alarm clock. These devices radiating through our bodies twenty-four seven are preventing us from activating our superpowers. The 5G, satellites, radiation, and signals all wreak havoc on our energetic bodies.

Never leave your computer on sleep. This allows access to your computer when you are away from it, which in turn can jeopardize your information, your bank accounts, and your computer files.

> ### JOURNAL: Chapter 7
>
> 1. What are your learning styles?
> 2. What new learning styles will you bring in?
> 3. What strategies do you want to incorporate into your life?
> 4. What ideas will you use when it comes to planning for your future?
> 5. What activity can you pick up that allows you to use both hands to access both parts of your brain?
>
> Keep writing in your gratitude journal every day!

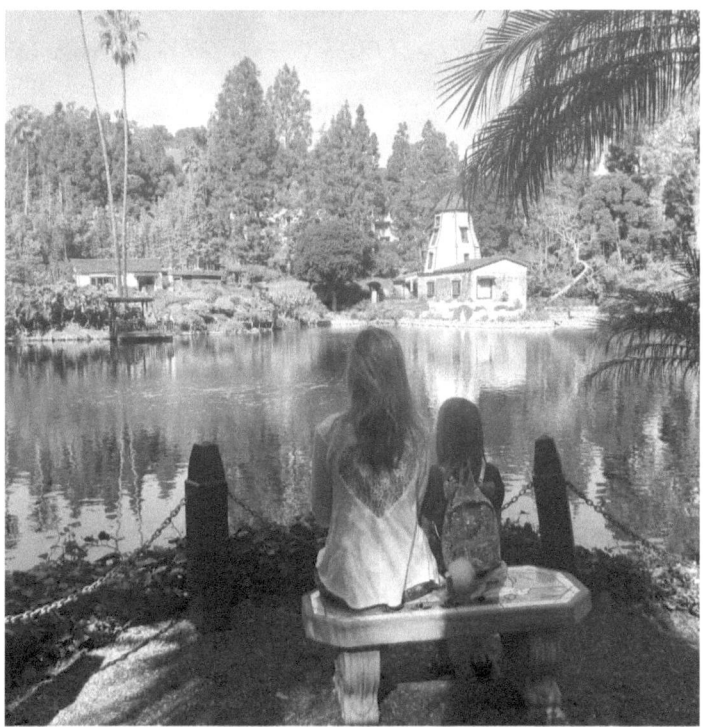

Here is a list of some books that changed my life in the meaningful ways:

- *To Fly Again* by Gracia Burnham with Dean Merrill
- *If I Could Raise My Kids Again* by William L. Coleman (parenting book)
- *Loyalty to Your Soul* by H. Ronald Hulnick and Mary R. Hulnick
- *The Little Book of Skin Care* by Charlotte Cho (girls, you are gonna love this)
- *The Purpose Driven Life* by Rick Warren
- *Protecting the Gift* by Gavin De Becker (keeping kids and teens safe)
- *The Gift of Fear* by Gavin De Becker (survival signals that protect us)

- *The Four Agreements* by Don Miguel Ruiz
- *The Top Ten Things Dead People Want to Tell You* by Mike Dooley
- *The Celestine Prophecy* by James Redfield
- *The Artist Way's* by Julia Cameron
- *Calling in the One* by Katherine Woodward Thomas
- *The Psychic Pathway* by Sonia Choquette

## Practice Checks

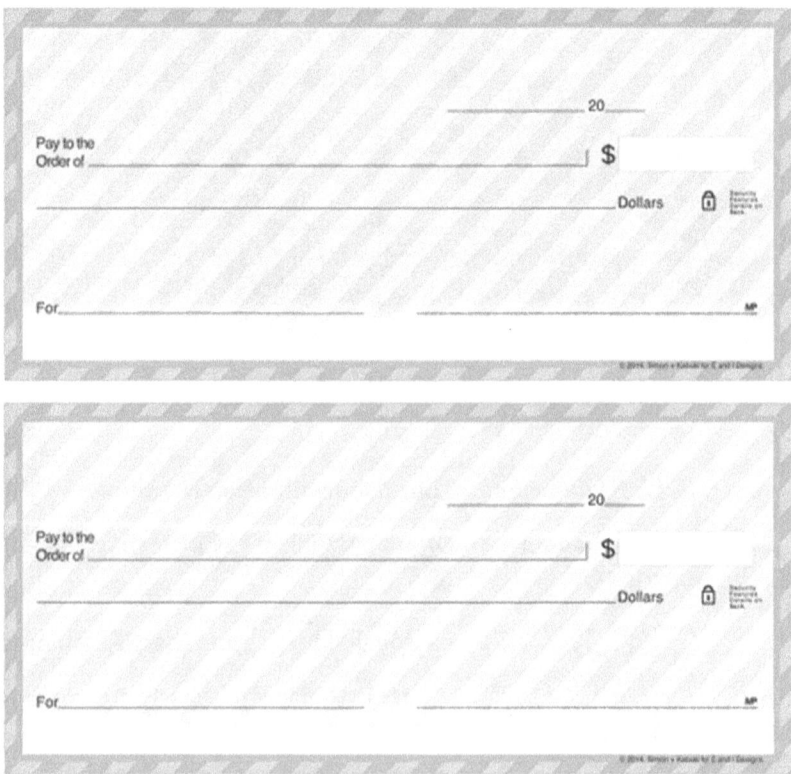

# CHAPTER EIGHT

# DNA

We need to monitor our DNA and our kids' DNA. This is how we can determine our soul purpose, our true path, what we like, what we are good at, and where we should put our attention and energy.

As adults, we tend to push our desires, morals, values, and ethics on our children. In some cases, this is a good thing—in others, not so good. Each person has their own blueprint in the universe and on this planet, which needs to be honored in order for them to thrive.

Our DNA needs to be studied and protected. Why? Because we are facing so many pollutants in food, drugs, vaccines, water, air, etc. Our DNA is our lineage and heritage and carries a lot of information. It is passed down from one generation to the next. If it gets mutated and messed up, that can impact the future of mankind.

## STUDY YOUR DNA

In my lifetime I have discovered ways to study my DNA and blueprint as well as my kids'. And I am going to share that with you. I have been told all my life what to believe and how to behave, and I was unsupported in the choices I have made because society doesn't deem them acceptable. I think outside the box. It's the way I'm genetically made—unique just like you. I discovered my type of personality makes up only 2 to 3 percent of the population, which can make it really hard to fit in. I am operating, thinking, and vibrating at a different level than most, though we all still vibrate as one.

My job is to bring the future to you, just like Elon Musk and Nicolas Tesla. Many people consider Elon Musk a nutjob, when in reality that man is so ahead of our time that many people can't begin to comprehend his genius. These pooh-poohers are of an old-school, limited mindset. We have been presented with a lot of hypotheses about the future via TV, films, and books. Films I want you to check out: *Escape from New York*, *Total Recall*, *The Terminator*, *Avatar*, *The Matrix*, *Xanadu*, *Star Wars*, *Star Trek*, and the *Left Behind* series. You may have seen and heard of these, but watch them again. Watch them after you read this book and see if you pick up new information.

The TV shows my eleven-year-old daughter is watching in 2022 are talking about chakras, energy, decisions, and strategies, so I know it is time for me to present this information without fear of being judged and rejected. It is time for everyone to wake up and be open to the invisible, the unknown, and the unbelievable. Also check out the film *The Adam Project* with Ryan Reynolds. These films could be made up, or they could be preparing us for what is to come.

## Heritage/Lineage

From research, I've discovered that fears, values, beliefs, morals, viewpoints, and the like can be passed down from generation to generation. What happened in your lineage has carried down to you.

Centuries and millennia ago, when someone got bit by a venomous spider, they didn't have a hospital to go to, and there was no cure, so people would die from spider bites. Today, many people are afraid of spiders and don't know why. The truth is that someone in their bloodline had a traumatic experience with spiders. I believe it could very well be tied into our unconscious and subconscious mind as well.

## Past Lives/Reincarnation

I have always believed in reincarnation. We might not remember anything, but who says our subconscious and unconscious mind or DNA doesn't? The human body is a complex organism that we are still trying to understand. Its expansion can be infinite.

When I was in my mid-forties, a young woman who I had been friends with for a while asked me to have a foursome with her, her boyfriend, and her girlfriend. They were all roommates in their early twenties. I was flattered but knew I would never be able to get intimate with other people that way. (My soul is only compatible one true, pure connection.)

I asked her, "Do you think you are a man in a woman's body?"

And without hesitation she replied, "Yes, absolutely."

You see, back when I was growing up, being gay, lesbian, and bisexual was not considered okay, to a much larger degree than today. Many parts of society still use religion to control people's sexuality. Parents shun their children, turn them away, or cut them off. It is a very hard passage for people who prefer a partnership that is not accepted by those who have power over them. Kids often don't tell their parents.

In my soul, I've long known that people are being reincarnated into bodies of different genders, which confuses the soul when it comes to determining which gender it feels like and which it should prefer. Think about it: if you were a woman in lifetime after lifetime, and then suddenly you came into this world as a man, it would be a shock. Your body parts would be different, but your brain, soul, conscious, subconscious mind, and unconscious mind would tell you otherwise.

This to me explains why so many people are becoming more fluid when it comes to sexual preference and self-identification. TV shows are acknowledging and incorporating LGBT, gays, lesbians, etc., and it's about time. Now, your parents or grandparents may not accept this, because they don't understand; let me remind you: beliefs are passed down from generations. But if you are gay or however you define yourself, it is perfectly okay. Each of us has a different experience when it comes to our sex life, based on experiences, past lives, and upbringing. I am here to remind you to do what is right for you.

Do not let others dictate how you should think, feel, or behave. You are you. Hone it and own it.

I was involved with a very religious man who didn't believe in reincarnation and chakras and was against gays and very into Christianity. This has been the mindset of many people on this planet for generations. I was met with this kind of resistance for many years. He missed the entire point and just drew up conclusions based on his upbringing. There is a very good chance you might face the same circumstances in your family.

I believe divorce is caused by differences in belief systems surfacing years and even decades after marriage, with each spouse now refusing to accept the other for who they are. That is why it is so important to choose a partner who is in alignment with your beliefs, values, and viewpoints to a certain extent. Otherwise you may face a head-on collision.

## Luminary Film

In 2014, I made a film dedicated to reincarnation called *Luminary*, and it is about the light within that we radiate out to the world: moments of time, moments of beauty, moments of magic, glimpses of who we are—all told through music, sound, energy, vibration, and no words. This is the way to truly communicate with each other as one.

When writing this book, I was moved to realize that everything I have been doing all my life has been geared toward the future and this book. The film has never been released, but the trailer is linked on my website. I hope to release the film right around the time this book drops. I invite you to watch my film trailer for *Luminary* at https://LuminaryHealingCenter.com under the media/appearances tab.

In 2018, I bought the domain name LuminaryHealingCenter.com, kept it for a year, then let it go. The idea was to open a healing center in order to share the healing modalities in this book to the public. Then COVID surfaced, and I put my plans on hold. Synchronicity hit when I went back a few years later and the domain name was still available. That is when I knew that this work is my soul purpose mission.

• • •

## WHAT IF?

What if we were all are from different planets in galaxies far, far away, brought to Earth to come together, mate, and coexist? What if we are currently living in a video game matrix that we define as the real world and our true bodies are somewhere else?

Sounds kinda scary. But would you do things differently? Would you search for who you are and master the game?

What would you do?

## NUMEROLOGY

Call me weird if you want, but I dream in numbers, and I see sequences. I believe it's yet another one of my superpowers rising.

Math and numbers are a universal language; species in different galaxies could communicate through numbers. Each number has a vibrational meaning attached to it, and when you combine numbers, you get a sequence of meanings. It's a pretty powerful tool that works in conjunction with everything around you. Your subconscious and unconscious mind pick up data constantly, even when you are sleeping; being mindful of your surroundings is imperative.

Numerology is an instrument used to explore our soul's blueprint. It focuses a spotlight on our greatest assets on the physical, emotional, mental, and spiritual planes. Numerology reveals our unique talents in order to help us gain a better understanding of ourselves and others. It can direct someone to the career choice that will best complement the personality code given to them, creating the opportunity to become more aware of their talents and path and of their compatibility with others.

Each number is influenced by a different planet in our solar system, including Pluto. Here we go again, looking out at space and the planets. Notice a recurring theme? Each letter of the alphabet vibrates to a given number, one through nine. Letters make up our names, giving us additional coding. These are just some of the tools we can use in working toward our mission in life and through all our karmic lessons. Numerology prompts insight into our self and others and wisdom. It is actually quite remarkable when you think about it and incorporate it into your life.

Just as your name carries vibrational meanings attached to numbers, so does your home address. That is why house buyers in certain cultures look at addresses before they even consider purchasing a property.

Here is a brief synopsis of what the numbers in numerology mean:

- 0: sign of eternity, evolution, and infinity since it looks like a circle. "God" force and universal energies. Reinforces, amplifies, and magnifies the vibrations of the numbers it appears with.
- 1: Sun planet; fiercely independent, competitive, determined, values freedom, original, leadership qualities, self-reliant. Ones can accomplish whatever they set their minds to. New beginnings, creativity, willpower.
- 2: Moon planet; inspiration and intuitiveness. Gentle and forgiving, trusting, has faith. Two is the most feminine among all numbers. Teamwork and relationships. Partnerships, trust, choices, balance.
- 3: Planet Jupiter; creativity, communication, optimism, curiosity. Triad, i.e., things in threes: past-present-future, birth-life-death, mind-body-soul. Mastery, completion, advancement.
- 4: Planet Uranus; solid, stable, and confident. Dislikes change, extremely dependable. Hard work, achievement, stability.
- 5: Planet Mercury; associated with the senses we have. These people are usually very beautiful and have a charismatic aura. They are quite fun loving, zealous, and cheerful. Adventure, passion, exploration.

- 6: Planet Venus; perfection and completion. People who have this number in their names are said to be trustworthy, dependable, and charming. Unconditional love, the ability to support, nurture, and heal. Growth, learning, protection.
- 7: Planet Neptune; deep and wise. Researcher, listener, sensing, search for awareness. Intelligent, analytical, powerful intuition. Shines a light into the very deepest realms to access hidden truths. Spirituality, mysticism, healing.
- 8: Planet Saturn; authority, self-confidence, inner strength, inner wisdom, social status, ego; love for humanity and a desire for peace. Extremely professional and very successful, especially in business. New opportunities, good fortune, abundance.
- 9: Planet Mars; represents completion, wisdom, and experience, and contains the energy both of endings and of new beginnings. Humanitarian, lots of love, accepting. Initiation, months spent in the womb.
- 10: attainment of greatness. New beginnings, leadership, confidence; independent, creative, success, energetic.
- Master numbers: numbers so important that they align with the three stages of creation.
    - ☐ 11: powerful intuition, seer, sensitive, works well with others, spiritual, cooperation, influence, instinct. Deep sense of awareness about the things we cannot see.
    - ☐ 22: master builder. Hard worker, confident. Powerful manifester, turns ideas into reality. Suffers setbacks to stay on track.
    - ☐ 33: master teacher. Purity, love, light, healing, enlightenment. Suffers heartache and hardship to show the way to hope and healing for others.

https://www.Numerology.com is a great site to check out.

I love reading license plates. There are some really creative ones out there. But when driving, I have to be careful not to pick up too much data, or all those numbers will start running around in my head. I try to be very aware of the info I allow to enter my personal mind database, as it influences my every move.

## ASTROLOGY

I don't know why people are so closed to astrology; perhaps they don't have the slightest clue who they are or what it is all about. Their mind is not expanded, so they miss out on seeing the benefits.

There is much more to astrology than your sun sign. Think of it like this: you come out of your mom on your birthing day at a given date, time, and location. Consider this your longitude and latitude in the universe. It reveals where the other planets were positioned relative to you at the moment of your birth. Where those planets are during your lifetime impacts the way you function. As the planets move, you move in certain directions and have certain experiences. If we pay attention, we can prepare for and understand what happens to us.

In astrology, each of the planets represents a different set of qualities and characteristics that rule over a different part of our lives—each bringing with them their own unique vibe and directive. You can think of the planets as characters, each with different goals, interests, and jobs.

Here is a breakdown of the planets and their meanings:

- Sun = ego
- Moon = emotions
- Mercury = communication
- Venus = love and relationships
- Mars = physical energy
- Jupiter = luck
- Saturn = structure

- Uranus = innovation
- Neptune = inspiration
- Pluto = rebirth

Tip: A great site to go to get a complete readout of your planet chart is https://www.astro.com. You can then go to YouTube and type in, say, "moon in Virgo," and videos describing related personality traits will come up. Break it down planet by planet, and you can learn a lot about yourself or someone else.

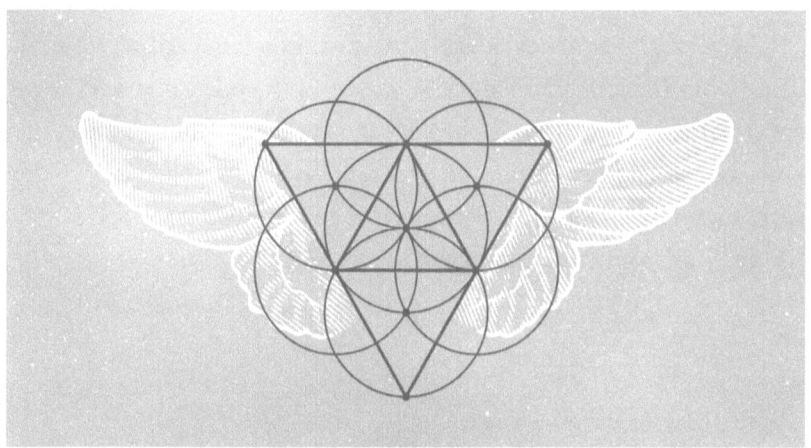

## SACRED GEOMETRY

Remember how I could do math in my head from a young age? Well, I have always been drawn to hexagons, triangles, and geometric shapes, which eventually led me to learn about sacred geometry. Sacred geometry attributes sacred meanings to certain geometric shapes and distinct patterns, forms, ratios, and numbers throughout the natural world and is considered the architecture of the universe. The leaves or branches of a tree, the spiral of a snail's shell, or the pattern of a single snowflake are examples of sacred geometry in nature.

Sacred geometry contains high frequencies of energy and light that can activate, heal, awaken, and transform. The codes it contains can be brought out into the conscious mind to activate deep soul awakening and connection to our true divine essence. Once I connected to sacred geometry, I started noticing it everywhere. It goes back in history to ancient times. Sacred geometry has recently been connected to sound frequencies. Check out https://www.cymascope.com to learn about a new invention that allows us to visualize sounds.

## SYMBOLISM

Symbolism attaches ideas and meanings to natural objects. These objects, noticed organically, can send us coded messages if we are receptive to them. The objects can represent a thought, feeling, emotion, or state of mind and can represent other objects. We are surrounded by symbolism. We just have to know what to look for.

Here are some fun examples:

- Red rose = love and romance
- Rainbow = promise and hope
- Four-leaf clover = good luck or fortune
- Shopping cart image = online purchases

Symbolism is used in books, movies, nature, money, and can be something as simple as a coin on the floor or a feather in the air. To me, symbolism is connected to synchronies. The universe is speaking to you and guiding you. Are you paying attention?

## ANIMAL TOTEMS

A totem animal is an animal spirit guide believed to stay with you for life. Other guides might enter your life and try to grab your attention when you are open and aware, but totem animals hold huge significance and are very dominant in Native American traditions.

They are believed to help you connect with your higher self and communicate through telepathic frequency.

You may notice an unusual creature in your life. Owls, for instance, are seldom seen or heard. When you do notice an owl, you notice it because it is rare. They might show up when you are in need of wisdom and intuitive knowledge. Animals have something to say if you stop and listen. Sure, you might not know the language, but you can figure out the message. Sit down and meditate on animals and interpret what they are trying to tell you through their energy, vibration, and sound. You might be surprised what messages they send you and how they make you feel.

If I get hit with something over and over, I take notice and look up the meaning in books or online. I have been hit hard by dragonflies and butterflies during transformation, the Japanese beetle when struggling with abundance, and rats when I am in survival mode. It is amazing to discover the underlying meaning of spirit animals. These animals have been communicating to our ancestors for centuries, so there could be a connection to certain animals in your DNA.

May you never look at wildlife the same way again.

## HUMAN DESIGN

Okay, I am going to throw something into the mix that not everyone knows about. After all, that's the point of this book.

Human Design offers a blueprint that indicates how you are unique as a person and guides you to live in sync with who you are. It brings together the principles of the I Ching, astrology, Kabbalah, Hindu-Brahmin chakra system, and quantum physics into a system of logic. Remember what I said about looking at other countries, systems, and patterns? This is the key to tying us into one component. Your Human Design chart, also called a "body graph," is calculated using your birth date, time, and place to reveal your genetic design. Here we go right back into DNA. It's a holistic self-knowledge system. If we know ourselves holistically, we will know how to heal the body holistically. Get it?

There are five energy types: manifesters, generators, manifesting generators, projectors, and reflectors.

Human Design is science being set apart and broken down. The Human Design chart consists of twenty-six activations, thirteen planetary imprints, nine centers, thirty-six channels, sixty-four gates/hexagrams (there's the math again), six lines, and three levels of substructure.

We need more people on the planet to integrate this kind of knowledge. To master this valuable tool for human understanding takes years of experience and wisdom. I have to say, Human Design is one of my top choices for guiding our children toward understanding who they will become. It has been one of the most empowering activations of self-alignment for me. When you truly understand why you came to this planet and you put all the pieces together to manifest your soul's purpose, the entire universe shifts in your favor, and the world aligns.

Working with a Human Design master will excel, amplify, and align you to become the best version of yourself. The elements a Human Design master looks at are directly related to your DNA, your chakras, meridians, gateways, and organs. The complexity and magnitude is unlike anything we have seen before. Every family, human, and being should consider looking at this chart if they want to know their purpose and connect with the divine. It really is like getting an owner's manual for ourselves.

Remember, the internet is swarming with people trying to steal your data as well as your mind and body. I highly recommend if you are going to do any type of assessment, you work on a very secure computer and use all possible security measures to protect your personal information.

You can go here and take the assessment, but you are going to need a true master to fully comprehend your results: https://www.jovianarchive.com/Human_Design/What_is_it.

## GENE KEYS

Another great way to chart your DNA is using the gene keys system (https://www.Genekeys.com). It yields yet another treasure map to discovering who you are. It highlights astrological calculations and the Chinese I Ching, creating a profile and offering individual insights. The gene keys teach contemplation, inquiry, gentleness, and patience, and they tie into and complement Human Design.

• • •

## DISCOVERING WHO YOU ARE

To learn more about yourself, you might consider taking personality assessments.

By breaking down what you are good at, an assessment can highlight natural talents and passions and tell you where to direct your attention and energy. This will help you academically and throughout the rest of your life.

The assessments dig down to what drives you, excites you, and motivates you. And learning about your family, friends, partners, coworkers, and teachers is really neat too. People who want to build successful business teams use this kind of data to fill in the gaps and tap into everyone's superpowers. One superpower a group doesn't have can be gained by bringing on someone else who has that superpower. You can't be amazing at every single thing; nor would you want to be. There are just some things that don't interest you and are not in your DNA. In order to get to the next level, we all have to work together as one.

This is why you don't want to put other people down. They are here to be weird, unique, funky, genius, intelligent, calm, simple, or whatever term you know them by. We need what they bring to the table. We must accept and appreciate one another for who we are. Do not judge anyone, and be kind to everyone, because you don't know what superpower they hold for the benefit of this planet.

## Types of Personality Assessments

I am not going to call these tests. Who wants to take a test? Nope, we are assessing the situation. Remember: no judgment, just observation. This is how we learn to accept one another for who we are. We are going to see how people think, process, and perform based on the way they are genetically built.

Time to embrace, enhance, excite, and expand our superpowers.

When taking any assessment, don't overthink your answers. Your gut reaction is usually the most accurate. Even if you don't like the answers, there are no right or wrong ones. Be as truthful as possible to get an accurate reading, and describe yourself as you function in normal, everyday life.

Get a three-ring binder and put all your assessments in one place. This way you can track, refer back to, and keep all in one place your DNA, blueprint, and assessments.

Once again, I highly recommend that you work on a very secure computer and use all available means to protect your personal information.

## DISC Assessment

A form of this test has been used quite a bit to build teamwork, communication, and productivity in the workplace. DISC assessments are used worldwide in organizations ranging from government agencies and Fortune 500 companies to nonprofits and small businesses.

By learning this at a young age, you can build better relationships.

In a more modern version of this assessment called DiSC®, *D* stands for dominance, *I* for influence, *S* for steadiness, and *C* for conscientiousness. Everyone is a mixture of each style, but most people tend to fall into one or two main categories. According to one DISC validation study, the *S* personality type ("submission" in some versions) is the most common DISC style at the global level, making up 32 percent of the worldwide population.

You can take the DISC assessment here: https://www.discprofile.com/what-is-disc.

## Color Code

The color code identifies not only what you do but why you do it, allowing deeper insights into what makes you and those around you fly off the handle. Each person has a dominant color and a secondary color that tend to stand out.

- Reds need to be right and respected. They are strong leaders, love challenges, and are often the head of a company.

- Blues need to be appreciated, and they have strong integrity. They are focused on creating strong relationships of quality.

- Whites have kindness as their motto and need to be accepted and treated this way. Whites are logical, objective, and tolerant of others.

- Yellows love life, beauty, and creativity, social connections, and being positive and spontaneous. They like to have fun and be the life of the party.

Do you demonstrate traits like these? Do your siblings? Your friends or family?

You can take the color code here: https://www.colorcode.com/.

You can also go to YouTube and type in "color code blue," and there are videos providing more detailed descriptions and information on compatibility between the colors. See how useful this might be when choosing a partner to mate with for life?

There are apps that connect like-minded people based on these and other types of assessments, such as the app called the Pattern. Imagine yourself in the future, pulling out your phone to share extensive DNA knowledge and compatibility, blood type, and STD results with a potential partner. That is some pretty powerful info at the ready to help guide your next move. It's just a matter of time before it evolves beyond our current applications.

## Sixteen Personalities

Honestly, I think we all are filled with personalities. So many things come into play when we function that there is no way to be in control and aware of it all due to the subconscious and unconscious mind. You can get a "freakishly accurate" description of who you are and why you do the things you do by analyzing this aspect. You can also find out which celebrities have the same traits, which is pretty impressive.

I could break down all the personalities here, but I'd rather give you the link and let you have at it (discovery is part of the fun): https://www.16personalities.com/.

## Enneagram Personalities

The Enneagram of Personality is a model of the human psyche that is principally understood and taught as nine interconnected personality types. This system of personality typing describes patterns in how people interpret the world and manage their emotions. I will list them here so you can get the gist with the one-word descriptions: reformer, helper, achiever, individualist, investigator, loyalist, enthusiast, challenger, peacemaker.

Look around your classroom or workspace: do you see anyone who falls into some of these categories? What do you think you might fall under? You might be surprised when you take the assessment. Then again, you might have that aha moment, like, *Yes. I get it. That's me.*

Here is a link to take the assessment—https://www.personalitypath.com/free-enneagram-personality-test/—but feel free to find a link you may like better. Remember, you are in charge of your destiny and what feels right.

## Five Love Languages

As you grow up, you will hear more and more about this topic when it comes to choosing a mate. It is often brought to the forefront in online dating apps where people might express their languages in order of importance on their profile. What I have found is that if you don't have the same or similar love languages in the same order of importance, you don't have total alignment. What is important to you may not be important to your potential mate—which means the other person won't give you what you need to have in a thriving relationship. There will always be something missing.

Do yourself a favor and take the assessment and keep your love languages in mind. You are going to want to use them when choosing a partner. This type of information was missing years ago. But today, you will have it at the ready as part of your superpower knowledge.

These are the five love languages:

1. Words of affirmation: compliments/appreciation
2. Physical touch: physical gestures
3. Quality time: undivided attention
4. Acts of service: offering a service of value
5. Receiving gifts: symbols of thought

Five love languages assessment link: https://www.5lovelanguages.com/.

## Journal: CHAPTER 8

1. What personality assessments will you access to learn about your superpowers?
2. Watch the trailer for the film Luminary. How did it make you think and feel about reincarnation?
3. How do you feel about numbers? Sacred geometry? Symbolism?
4. Do you have a spirit animal? Which one would it be?

Keep the gratitude attitude going in your gratitude journal!

Don't forget to print and put your assessments in a binder to refer back to anytime. You will be surprised how many similarities show up in due time.

Make binders for each of your kids, creating their very own adventure guide storybook.

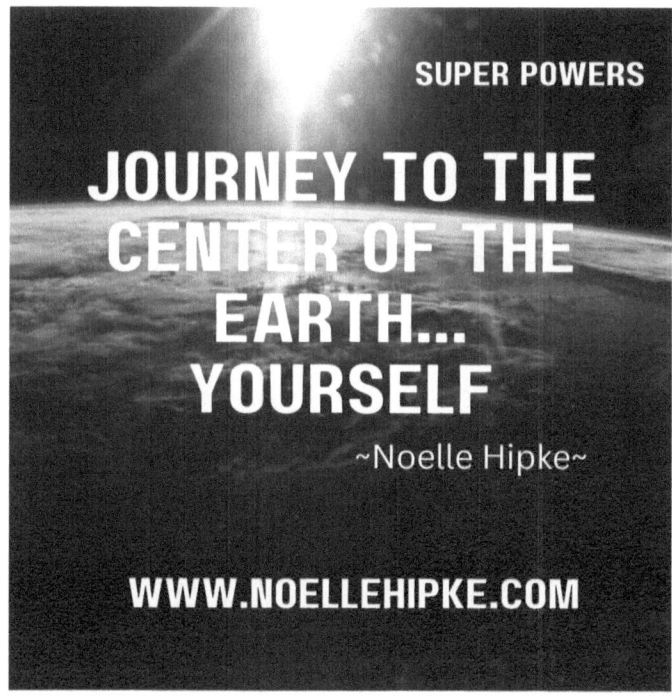

## CHAPTER NINE

# HEALING THE BODY

My entire fifty-one-year journey has been devoted to healing the body and soul. I want to show you ways you can heal the body all on your own. I believe when you heal the soul, you elevate to a status that is beyond belief. Our ancestors, our kids, our parents, our brothers and sisters, and future generations are healed. We are all one in vibration, light, and sound. When you do the work to heal your soul, you elevate humanity.

Those are some pretty powerful superpowers we have. Only, no one ever talks about this. Why? Because they don't understand. The new earth is changing from a materialistic world to an energetic one. I am being divinely guided to share the knowledge of the future in the present moment so you all can elevate and transcend. I literally stopped my life to write this book, and I've poured my heart and soul into it. You are ready to receive and implement the information. Some of it may be brand new, but along the way, you have all been given glimpses—in movies, words, symbols, signs, songs, animals, nature, vibrations, energy, thought patterns, waves, and motion.

Holistic health is the path to healing the body, mind, and soul, as you will read in these last few chapters. I am so excited to bring this new-earth holistic healing concept out into the open. May your inner light shine to eternity. We are luminary.

## EXERCISE

I know a lot of you might not want to hear this, but exercise is one of the fountains of youth. It literally changes the cells in your body to jump-start your natural capabilities to heal. You need to get your blood pumping in order to flush out your system. This removes impurities in the body and creates collagen to build strong bones and boost elasticity of your skin and connective tissue. It also helps build healthy muscle, which will start to diminish as you get older. The main objective is to detox all the crap so the body has optimum health to eliminate waste and dead cells. Removing this material frees up your body to regenerate and revive.

In order to activate your superpowers, you need to make exercise part of your routine three to five times a week. Many people get addicted (in a good way) when they realize it gets their superpowers going.

When I was a kid, I hated physical education. None of us wanted to sweat and ruin our hair and makeup in PE. But that it is exactly what we need to do. Sweating out the poisonous toxins we ingest on a daily basis is vital, which is why I am putting it at the top of the list in this chapter. Our bodies and armpits reek for a reason: the toxins are getting out. Many of the yogis I've hung out with never would wear antiperspirants, which often contain aluminum and other toxins that can cause health issues. Centuries ago, all were stinky. Learn to love yourself when you smell.

You can buy deodorant that doesn't contain toxins, but learn to read labels, and ask your body, *Is this the right product for me?*

### Running

Some days I got so worked up from the mental and physical abuse in my home that I would go outside and run until I could no longer stand up. I would drop in place, panting and breathing heavily with tears streaming down my face. I needed to release the energy and stress my body was holding on to. I didn't care who saw me.

I had no idea at the time why I did it. My body just told me to do it, and I listened. And this is what I want you all to do. Tune in to your body. Only you know your body and what is right for you. If it's walks and yoga, go do it. Ride a bike, swim, do a sport. Hit it hard. Your body will tell you. All you have to do is listen. So go out, move, and sweat. It's a great way to get away from all these stupid electronic devices and align with yourself, your vibration, your energy.

## Gym

I go to the gym for classes and personal workouts, though exercising outside is the best option if you live in an environment with fresh, clean air. Often I ride my beach cruiser along the boardwalk, getting sunshine and vitamin D—I call this the happiness workout. It elevated my mood, and the awesome tunes I played in my headphones brought my vibration to another level.

Exercise and music can have a powerful healing effect on the body when intertwined. You can remember good times with a familiar song, or create an entire new vision of life in your head with music you have never heard before. You are programming your brain to feel happiness and positivity and aligning your cells to create anything you want. By envisioning it, feeling it, and believing it, we create it.

There have been times at the gym when I'm riding the bike and I cross this threshold where I get into the zone and my body starts sweating. It's a sudden natural high. I have always wanted to film myself at this moment, as if I'm in a commercial, screaming, "Yes! Yes! Yes!" like a woman having an orgasm. I create the environment in my head and body to get into that state. Many times, it's hard to hold back. And now when I ride my bike outside in public, I start yelling, "Woo-hoo!" I pour good energy out to others as I ride by. Everyone smiles, laughs, and sometimes they yell back. Positive energy can be contagious.

So get your fanny outside and exercise, or do it inside—whatever it takes. Move the energy no matter what, make it part of your lifestyle, and you will reap the benefits for the rest of your life.

## Dancing

Dancing raises your vibration. By shaking my body all over to amazing music, I feel such love for myself. I feel good and free. I become one with the music, vibrate higher, and feel the cells in my body tingle when my body aligns with the frequency of the music tones. I become electric, unlimited, unstoppable. My mind shows me ways to do things better, and my body is excited to have the connection and attention, aligning me to higher frequencies, vibrations, and realms.

## Sprinklers

One night in my mid-forties, at 3:30 a.m. in Palm Springs, I was hanging out with friends on the golf course at a condo when the sprinklers came on. I got the sudden urge to run through them and yelled, "Let's run in the sprinklers like kids." And we did.

It was one of those beautiful, fun experiences I will remember for the rest of my life. It was magic. Water carries energy and vibration, and so does the earth and grass. We ran barefoot through the sprinklers like little kids. And you know what? I felt free and young like a little kid. And guess what the cells in my body were doing. Healing. Vibrating high like a kite naturally. We were connected to the water, the earth, and each other as one. We were magnificent beings activating our superpowers.

## Dancing in the Rain

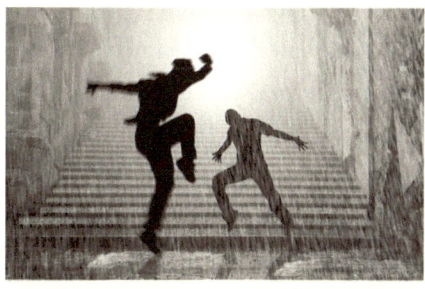

At one point, I didn't like the rain. My house had several leaks that didn't get fixed properly when I put on a new roof. Every time it rained, I would get upset, worried, and concerned. Then one day I recalled the amazing sprinkler experience from years earlier and made a pivotal turn.

From that moment on, I decided to embrace the rain. I put up tarps to fend off the leaks, and I grabbed my ten-year-old daughter and put a boom box at the backyard door. Wearing our pajamas in the rain, we played our favorite songs and we danced our butts off to the magic that was taking place around us. A celebration of life—the plant life, the nature life, animal life, and our life. We held hands and ran in a circle with the song "Just the Two of Us" blasting in the background, an oldie but goodie.

The electricity shared between two people holding hands in the rain is amazing. Your light and frequency become one. If you plug in an electrical cord and place it in water you are sitting or standing in, you get electrocuted and die. But we are special electrical beings when it comes to dancing in the rain. This shared frequency gave me access to the information floating around all of us. My senses were amplified, and I was elated beyond belief. I remember turning to my daughter to say, "When I am on my death bed, I want you to remember this." It was another one of the most beautiful moments in my life, and I made sure to imprint this on both of our brains.

From that day forward, we always danced in the rain. Even if I didn't feel like it, my daughter would drag me outside; she could help me change my energy from negative to positive in just a few moments. Rain is magic. You are magic. This is how you connect, create, and generate.

On my birthday in 2021, my daughter and I were in different places on the planet. It rained. I went out and danced in the rain, and so did she. A rainbow surfaced, and we shared the beautiful energy with each other, even separated as we were. I tell you this story so you never look at the rain the same again. I would love for you to get off the couch and take on this experience for yourself.

Activate your life force energy. Feel your magnificent superpowers. You are a beautiful being, at one with the earth and each other.

• • •

## FART

I have to tell you, when you are moving energy in the body, you are going to build up some gas. And you are going to want to let it out so you can move the energy through your body. This is how universal energy flow works.

When I attended yoga classes, people often farted in front of everyone. And that is a good thing. They were releasing stuck energy in their organs and body. I didn't understand this when I was younger because of the embarrassment factor, but I totally get it today. While writing this book, I've had to fart a lot to push the energy through the body. I have to laugh: this is probably why I remained single while writing this book. I would have been too embarrassed to fart and would have held it in.

Society tells you it's not okay to fart in front of others. Which means you are holding all that energy in, and it is getting stuck in your body. Yuck. We don't want to do that. Stuck energy causes illness. Run out of the room if you have to, and let that puppy out. I don't even try to hold them back anymore. I just let them rip. It helps that there are just girls in the house, but I have to say that it has been rather freeing. And now I don't think I could hold them in if I wanted to, knowing how much more important it is to let them out. I have now farted in front of other people and just ignore the fact. There is a very good reason why our bodies make sounds when they do things: they are releasing blocked energy.

## SHOWERS/BATHS

Water is healing life force. Water is cosmic energy. When you need to clear energy for yourself, take a warm bath with bath salts to help remove impure energy from your body. Just be aware that if the water is too hot, it will remove natural oils and dry out your skin.

I place a wireless speaker in the bathroom with happy music when

I shower and calming music when I take a bath, for two very different reasons. A bath is a slower, longer process of release and meditation. Envision the impurities going down the drain when you let the water out. When I shower, I use more of the high-frequency healing by playing upbeat music. The higher frequencies vibrate through the water to put me into a higher vibration state. Remember what I said about sound traveling five times faster through water? Well, think about what that is doing for your body when you have awesome music playing next to the shower.

Let's call it an automatic upgrade. And use deodorant without aluminum.

• • •

## JOURNAL

Never underestimate the power of journaling. When you write, you create and manifest. This is your higher self trying to communicate to you, through you, directly to you. Decades ago, the book *The Artist's Way* really helped trigger my need to write. It guides you to write first thing in the morning every day. It wants you to exercise your brain like a muscle, and by doing it right when you wake up, you are working with a clean slate.

I have journals all over my house. I have a journal for dreams, educational TV shows I watch, outlines for books I read, classes I've taken, webinars I've attended, and YouTube videos I like. When something pops into my head, I write it down. I have to get it out. It all helps me fine-tune to my higher self and equip myself with the tools I need to compose this book.

I should have realized in high school that I had a writer in me. The only people who knew it were my friends. I couldn't see my superpower because my family didn't acknowledge it. I've tried to write this book several times in my life, but when I shared my idea with my mother, she said, "Why would you do that? It's not going to pay the bills." Sound familiar to you artists out there? At this point, I don't care if it doesn't pay the bills; it's what lights me up and gets my superpowers flowing, so I know I'm on the right track.

If you follow your passions and communicate authentically, you will radiate the energy needed to attract the right people.

As I mentioned at the beginning of this book and in the section about depression, I recommend you get several blank notebooks from the dollar store. Use one to write down thoughts you just can't get out of your mind, another to pour out all that you are grateful for, and maybe one to release all the things that are eating at you. Removing the blocks and toxicity of negative thinking helps free the mind to allow higher healing frequencies to flow in.

Using paper journals frees you from the Wi-Fi, radiation, and online security issues.

Journaling tips:

- Journal when you want to change something.
- Journal when you want to alter your genetic imprint.
- Journal when you want to change your programming.
- Journal when you want to change beliefs.
- Journal to create your own book.

## Gratitude Attitude

My daughter came up with the term "gratitude attitude" one evening when I was leading a vision board class. We all loved the term and started using it everywhere all the time. When one of us needed to be reminded we were getting out of alignment, someone would say, "Gratitude attitude," and we would immediately stop what we were doing and reflect to remember what we were thankful for. It is a great way to catch ourselves and redirect our thought patterns and remember what is really important.

I am always thanking people for their time and energy. I remember thanking the dentist after he ripped out my dental bridge. He was floored. Most people who go to the dentist don't want to be there. The dentist can feel our negative energy about the uncomfortable situation. Did you know dentists have one of the highest suicide rates? I do believe all this negative energy radiating from patient to doctor is the main factor. When I thanked him, he practically fell off his chair. He lit up. What he does is really important to humanity, but most people don't think of it this way. Realize that the people who take really good care of you are your cheerleader advocates. If someone doesn't come across the right way to you, move on to the next. You will see and feel the difference when a caregiver is genuine and sincere. The more they resonate with you, the better type of healer they are for you.

## Vision Boards

I have been doing vision boards for many years. Vision boards are created by taking photos, words, graphics, and a combination of other art ideas and placing them on a poster board. I typically use magazines, computer printouts of things I can't find organically, or words, stickers, gemstones, and other objects to make them three dimensional. I love seeing my goals, visions, affirmations, ideas, feelings, and dreams on my board. I include places I want to go, good health, relationships I'd like to have, and careers I would like to pursue. I even attach my board to a special custom picture frame. It hangs like art right next to my bed so I can look at it every night before I go to bed and first thing when I wake up in the morning. I get reminded multiple times a day about what is important to focus on for me and my family.

The creativity that pours out of me when composing these boards is endless, often taking me days to complete. I keep the boards so I can review them years later to see whether what I tried to manifest has lined up. Things don't always happen right away; that is the beauty with the timing of the universe. There are lessons you are supposed to learn along the way in order for you to truly accomplish your desires.

I decided to start hosting a vision board class in my garage with friends. The day of the event, I had no idea how I was going to lead them. Then, as if by magic, the ideas flooded in. I came up with a theme, a song, energetic exercises, a meditation, and the event flowed without a hitch, as did the ones that followed. My daughter joined us at the age of eight to make what may have been her third vision board. She had watched me make them over the years and took the initiative to make them on her own when she was looking for something fun to do. Her earlier boards included makeup, art, design, and fashion clothing, while this one included constellations, planets, and nature. This is when she came up with the term "gratitude attitude."

You will get some of your best insights by creating your vision and then going out to make it happen. Never underestimate the power of you.

. . .

## TELEVISION

As I've mentioned, I avoid TV news and all the negativity it brings, as well as the people who insist on filling me in on what I missed. I have felt their fear, heard it in their voices, and separated myself from people who vibrated like this. All that jibber jabber prevented me from listening and trusting myself and using my superpower survival skills to pick up on vibrational frequencies giving me the messages I really needed to hear from around the world. That is how you get in true alignment with yourself. You have to go deep within and listen.

I have disconnected from everything to compose this book. The world is on mute so I can hear my true higher self. I discovered when I completely let go and go within, I get all the messages I need to fly high naturally.

The only way to truly heal our bodies is to shut out the news, social media, and negative people. The pandemic can generate panic or it can generate self-healers, survivors who have activated their superpower instincts by going within to heal themselves.

## LISTEN UP

In my early fifties, I got caught up watching a TV show on a channel that had commercials. I hardly watch shows anymore that have commercials, but in order to access some old films, you have to use TV apps, and many times they have commercials to cover the cost.

It's almost like the app knew my age group and what I was concerned about. It presented a commercial that was about laundry detergent, but the emphasis it placed on wrinkles was ridiculous. I can't tell you how many times it said wrinkles in the commercial. Wrinkles this, wrinkles that. It wasn't really about the wrinkles on the clothes as much as it was conveying that no one wants to have wrinkles. I remember noticing and saying, "I caught you." These subliminal messages are coming in constantly, feeding the brain and changing our chemistry to believe them. Yuck. This is really quite frightening when you think about it.

And the amount of prescription drug commercials directed to senior citizens that air during the shows they most likely watch, such as *Jeopardy* and *Wheel of Fortune*, is insane. Many pharmaceutical companies in the United States only have their own interests at heart. They want to make you think about taking their drugs to fix your problems so they can make money, control you, or manipulate your body and DNA. The bad side effects listed in commercials often outweigh any good coming out of it.

People are diagnosed with mental issues and given drugs to numb them. What if these people are just more tapped into their superpowers than others? Yet they are immediately told they should not be feeling a certain way. People, parents, and doctors might sweep the real problem under the rug: perhaps healing emotions need to be addressed, or extrasensory abilities are picking up data that most people can't access.

What about addressing the real issue here? What if they are in a bad situation they need to get out of, and their body is just responding to the situation to get them to take notice and make a shift? What if they are eating the wrong foods for their body, they are in a toxic environment, or they have been exposed to a cleaning chemical that is causing a reaction? So many things can come into play. But the first thing most people do is turn to a drug. Huh?

Get off all medications. Go natural high. Exercise and put healthy food in the body, and you are ahead of this game. Think of it like a video game if you have to.

• • •

## PODCASTS

I'm repeating myself in this book, but that means you are supposed to hear it more than once. How else are you going to internalize all this good data? I have been listening to podcasts for years and attending events with podcasters. In 2014 I attended the National Association of Broadcasters (NAB) Tradeshow in Las Vegas, Nevada. According to Wikipedia, NAB is a "trade association and lobby group representing the interests of commercial and non-commercial over-the-air-radio and television broadcasters in the US." I learned about NAB in the broadcast journalism college class I was taking in 2014. Students got a hefty discount to attend, and I took up the offer.

These trade shows offered enhanced training and the latest technologies coming to the market. I was exposed to drones and phone gimbals in 2014 before they hit the public forum. Podcasting was just starting to hit the market, and I was considering this up-and-coming profession. Who knows, maybe I will go there someday.

I've always loved learning from others. I spent days at the event, learning and talking to anyone who would offer me insights. I was invited to attend private events, hang out with the elites, and was granted access to listen to famous speakers and film producers. It was an incredible opportunity to make connections.

## Podcasters

A few years later, I went on a date with a guy named Brian Scott who is on YouTube and also has a podcast, called *The Reality Revolution*. At the time, he shared that he'd had a near-death experience, which accelerated his awareness process. He was at a vibrational frequency level I could not quite comprehend yet. Everyone is on different levels on this journey, just like in a video game, but we are all interacting together as one.

When we met, he had about 25,000 followers on his YouTube channel. Today, it's around 500,000. On his podcast, he reads chapters of books well beyond most people's comprehension. I remember calling and telling him, "These podcasts are way too long. You need to make them shorter." They were over an hour, and I was looking for smaller segments that contained the same info since it took so much concentration to interpret. Brian said, "No. I am being directed to do it this way." I accepted his reasoning and continued to listen.

Once you really listen, there are hidden nuggets in there. I loved the messages, data, and vibrations he was sending out. And if I didn't get a chance to finish the podcast, I would go right back into them when I could. He and the writers he reads from have received insights that are ahead of their time, and I realized he was put in my life so I could learn from him. He helped propel me into new areas I had not seen or understood before. In fact, when looking back at my life, I see that every single experience was meant to get me to this exact point in my life to put in on paper for you.

Great podcasters to check out:

- *The Melissa Ambrosini Show* (Australia)
- *The Reality Revolution* with Brian Scott
- *Raising Daughters* with Tim Jordan, MD

- *Doctor Thyroid* with Philip James
- *Dr. Wayne Dyer* (Hay House)
- *Love Life* with Matthew Hussey
- *Super Soul* with Oprah
- *Impact Theory* with Tom Bilyeu
- *You Can Heal Your Life* (Hay House)
- *Ted Talks Daily*
- *Powerful Ladies* (Orange County, CA)
- *The Ed Mylett Show*
- *The Rachel Hollis Podcast*
- *It's a Good Life* with Brian Buffini
- *Highest Self Podcast*
- *Earn Your Happy* with Lori Harder
- *Don't Keep Your Day Job* with Cathy Heller
- *Earth Speak* with Natalie Ross
- *SoulTalk* with Kute Blackson
- *Happiness Podcast* with Dr. Robert Puff, PhD
- *Expanding Reality*

• • •

## AUDIOBOOKS

I also love audiobooks. I can learn anything I want from any book that sparks my interest, and I don't have to be sitting down. You can put your phone in a booty bag with corded headphones and multitask the world around you. I've spent many of my days with an audiobook running in the background.

I love audio learning. Doing things while listening to the right content programs good things in your head. Get a couple audiobooks on anything you have ever wanted to learn, and you are ahead of the game. This helps you figure out the rules—since no one gave us any rules or manuals at birth.

## YOGA

When I was fourteen, my dad lived in Hawaii, and we kids went over for the summer. I now realize my dad was spiritual and my mother is not. You might have grown up in a similarly conflicted home. My dad was intuitive, had photographic memory, was creative, fun, loving, a freedom seeker and boomerang hucker, welder, marketer, and Harley Davidson rider in the 1970s. That man could create, figure out, and fix anything on the planet. He built an entire addition on our home without a construction background. He was also highly sensitive.

I truly believe a lot of alcohol and drug addicts and even people in insane asylums are hugely sensitive. They are told it is not okay to feel their feelings. In turn they try to bring down these emotions with drugs and alcohol and fall in line—do what everyone else who is normal does. That is total crap. We are not all the same. Why would we all act and try to be the same?

So, anyway—got on another rant there—my dad decided to sign me up for yoga classes while I was staying in Hawaii. That was one of those aha moments. Picture me lying on the grass under palm trees in the Hawaiian sun on a yoga mat under the blue sky. The palm trees are swaying, and I can hear the wind flowing through the fronds. It is utter magic.

Pay attention to your magic moments; those are the memories you will want to use later to help duplicate the feeling. If fact, write down your best memories in another journal so you can turn to them when you need to. I believe you should start doing yoga at a young age so you can learn about yourself and your body. Yoga brings you into deep connection and alignment with yourself. In turn, you will get more messages about what you and your body need from life. Yoga should be offered in PE in high school and students given the option to instruct if they are inclined to do so.

Yoga connects you to your higher self and source.

• • •

## MEDITATION

Meditation should be a part of your life forever. As I've said, shutting out the outside world is a great way to hear and align with your higher self. Ask yourself a question, and then go into a meditation to find the answer. You have the universe inside of you; this is how you access it. Do you get it? It's like we are typing the question into our personal computer and accessing our own database without outside influences. People who say they can't meditate can't hear themselves. They follow and do what everyone else is doing, but they do not understand the true purpose.

Meditation raises your vibration and enables universal energy flow to move through you, which allows you to connect to other vibrations and frequencies in order to gain knowledge. Universal energy flow exists on a higher vibrational frequency than we do physically here on earth. You need to raise your vibration to connect with it in order to reap the unlimited benefits, potentials, and portals. This is where you will get some of your most enlightened messages.

You can also listen to a meditation to get into the habit. Meditation is medication for the body. There are so many great meditations out there. Insight Timer is one of the best apps around—no commercials, great content from people around the world. It offers talks, meditations, music, guided imagery, yoga *nidra* (activating and thanking each body part, i.e., superpower gratitude activation), and much more as it adds healers and incredible wisdom sharers from around the world.

## Guided Imagery

When I was a little girl, around eight years old, I had a best friend who was an only child. Her parents loved me and treated me better than their own child at times. As a kid with two siblings, I gladly accepted that attention. They owned their own business, smoked illegal pot, and spoiled the heck out of us. We used to play office with their home business supplies, they took me to Disneyland, and I slept over at their house almost every weekend. I will never forget going through the McDonald's drive-through so they could get burgers to feed their dogs. Who does that? They were very much hippies living their own lifestyle in the moment.

One night, the mom put on a guided-imagery meditation for us to listen to as we dozed off. It guided us to envision ourselves by a stream of water in a garden and to walk around and look at the trees, the rocks, the flowers. It was pure, intentional, visionary meditation. I absolutely loved it. I looked forward to going over to her house to spend the night just so I could hear it. So, at a very young age, I was exposed to bits and pieces that helped me evolve to the person I am today. I was inadvertently programming my brain for the better in the 1970s. What are you doing today to program your brain for the better?

As my daughter grows, I continue to put on guided imagery, meditations, and healing music in the background as she falls asleep. This way I can program her brain to send and receive good thoughts, good vibrations, and happy feelings. This is how we tap into the subconscious and unconscious mind. But be very careful and selective with what you use. Remember me saying YouTube shows negative commercials in the middle of the night? I would put on a Disney Music kids meditation, and in the middle of the calming piano session, a commercial would come on full blast.

Record yourself on a device and play it back to your kids when they go to sleep. You can read a book or affirmations for your children to hear directly from you. We can never tell our kids enough how awesome they are, how proud of them we are, or how much we love them. Make this a habit, and I swear you will see a difference in how they operate, think, and feel about themselves.

## Fly or Invisibility?

Have you ever been asked to hypothetically choose between the superpower of flight or invisibility? Well, I want you to know we already have both. All we have to do is create it in our mind and leave our bodies behind, just like little kids do. We might have left our imaginations at the door when we grew up, but the possibilities are endless. We are unlimited. We can direct our minds to feel like we are flying and travel wherever we want to go. And if you want to be invisible, imagine that too, and people will ignore you. You will vibrate at a frequency that will not attract attention if you focus on creating it.

We can create anything we want. Do you understand and see that now? You can create the life you want by visualization and moving out of the physical body.

. . .

## AFFIRMATIONS

I love affirmations. Always have, always will. I have affirmations and reminders on sticky notes all over my house. How else are you going to remind yourself how amazing you are and to step up and improve? I tape them up in the bathroom so my daughter and I can be reminded every morning about what's truly important in life: Who am I? What is my purpose? What am I grateful for? I also have a map of consciousness, which describes feelings with words and gives each a vibrational frequency a level ranking. When I'm not feeling so good, or when I'm feeling the exact opposite, I walk in and look for my feeling on the chart to see what vibrational frequency I'm sending out. You can find that chart in the book *Power Vs. Force* by David R. Hawkins,

MD, PhD. Examples of frequency levels include enlightenment (700 to 1,000), peace (600), joy (540), anger (150), fear (100), guilt (30), and shame (20). It's an epic way to monitor and gauge yourself and how others are emitting.

Affirmations become second nature. They imbed in the brain. Every time I need something imbedded into my brain, I write it down and post it up. If I really need it to sink in, I say it out loud or yell it over and over.

I even record my affirmations and listen to them when I walk my dog around the block, fold laundry, water plants, and do the dishes. Those babies are going to stick. If you repeat something over and over, eventually it sinks in. Add some physical activity, and you are doing accelerated reprogramming on yourself.

• • •

## SOUND HEALING

The benefits of sound healing are extraordinary. And do traditional doctors use it? Nope. Notice a pattern here? Many aspects of holistic health are missing in our everyday healthcare in the US. Yet there is nothing traditional about healing the body. There is no one size fits all. So when they try to put you on a pill or medication, run for the hills unless you really need it to live. And if so, incorporate it slowly and remove yourself gradually when the time is right. You have to be in charge of your own health.

The body is an incredible self-correcting, self-healing organism. It just needs the proper tools. Each of you is unique, so your healing patterns are going to be unique as well. Multiple healing modalities may be required to peel back the layers of conditioning and toxicity, but it can be done with effort and intention. I have healed myself many times.

Sound healing is when instruments are used over and around the body to put the cells in a high cellular vibration. When cells vibrate in unison, it's like they are dancing inside your bloodstream; deep cellular healing occurs, and messages come through while you meditate to the music and observe yourself and your body.

Hands down, I believe sound frequency is the way we will heal in the future.

What frequencies do for the body:

- Send messages
- Aid clarity
- Affect red and white blood cells
- Elevate and transcend
- Heal the body
- Send knowledge and wisdom
- Send visions
- Help create our intentions
- Manifest
- Heal the soul
- Heal organs
- Send feelings
- Create learning
- Change brain patterns
- Create body energy
- Allow astral travel
- Change biochemistry
- Invoke transformation

I have received ideas on topics to include in this book when I allow music to flow through my body for several days in a row. I use that time with sound to wrap my head around the concept and the best way to present it. Some of this information is pretty advanced, so it takes time to process it correctly. My goal is to give you the viewpoint you need to comprehend it collectively.

A lot of negative frequencies that didn't used to exist surround our bodies on a daily basis. They are invisible, unidentified, and overlooked. Don't let this be you. It is more imperative than ever that you spend time doing frequency healing for yourself.

## Sound Baths

What are sound baths? Sound evokes deep states of awareness and emotional releases. Practitioners use vibratory instruments like singing bowls, gongs, chimes, and drums to enter a deep meditative state. The vibrations massage the body to release tension and relax the nervous system. Brain waves synchronize with sound waves, taking you on a vibrational journey within, to a deeper state of consciousness. Many people fall asleep during a sound bath, while others observe or meditate.

I remember my very first sound bath. I was the last of forty people to enter, and they were giving away a free ticket to a yoga retreat that was worth about $200. The sound bath was an incredible experience. When the drum was played over me, I felt it vibrating from the top of my head to my feet like a wave of energy. When I sat up after the sound bath was over, I thought, *This is my new jam.* A little girl walked over to the instructor to pick a name for the winning ticket. I thought, *Pick me, pick me*. And would you believe that little girl ended up picking me? That was when I knew I was in the right place at the right time.

During another sound bath I attended, a dental bridge that was in my mouth bled the entire time. As I meditated, I got messages that the bridge was infected and that it had been wreaking havoc on my entire central nervous system for years. Teeth are connected to all the organs in the body. Two days later, I went and got that bloody, infected bridge out and started a healing journey that required several implants over time. That journey brought me to the hospital due to the severity and duration of the infection. So let me tell you, your body knows what you need and what to do. All you have to do is tune in.

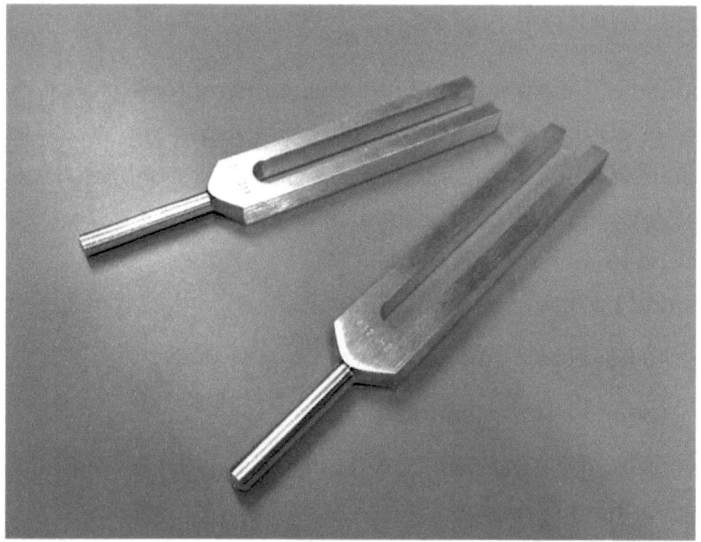

## Tuning Forks

These two-pronged metal forks are used as an acoustic resonator tool to tune musical instruments. However, breathwork guides and other healers have been using them on the body to disperse energy, relieve pain, and attune the body on a cellular level. I had a healer use them on me during a breathwork session, and hours later my body experienced a huge shift. I had been doing a lot of internal work, journaling, breathwork, and moving energy in the body; my body reacted with a panic attack from opening up a gateway that had not been cleared or activated for decades. That particular gateway connected me back to a precise day.

The session triggered a clearing connected to a day thirty-eight years prior, to the exact day my dad passed away. The tuning forks opened up and activated an internal portal, releasing years of pent-up energy. So much energy was moving and realigning that it caused chaos in my body for a short period. This can happen when you move too much energy in the body at one time or when working in deeper levels of the soul.

## Sound Journal Notes

Sound is the expression of universal mind source. Remember how sound travels through water five times better than air? Which means sound affects the baby in the womb, wiring its nervous system and organs. Imagine what kind of children we could raise if we orchestrated the sound healing they received.

Sound has many qualities:

- Sound can be music, speech, song, or prayers.
- Sound encodes information.
- Sound creates vibratory paths to parallel dimensions and brings knowledge.
- Many cultures put value on sound and the spoken word.
- Words have power. We manifest and influence by the words we speak.
- Sound is the key to higher realities and ourselves.
- The way through the matrix is to raise your vibration.
- Sound ties into mathematics, cell division, and sacred geometry.
- The whole universe is vibrational. What happens in us is reflected in the greater cosmos.
- Life is music with overtones.
- Forest sounds hold knowledge; respect and listen to nature.
- Particles and waves affect us.
- The universe is a cosmic symphony singing a song to the creator.

I want you to be aware that sounds online can be tampered with and may not come from pure intentions. Be very careful about the channels you listen to. I remind you, sound is the expression of universal mind source. If that source is looking to control you, it may very well be done through sound.

## TELEPATHY

During my divorce, I started detoxing the body, eating healthier, fasting, exercising, and working on myself. I was moving in a new direction, and so was my body. New superpowers started to appear.

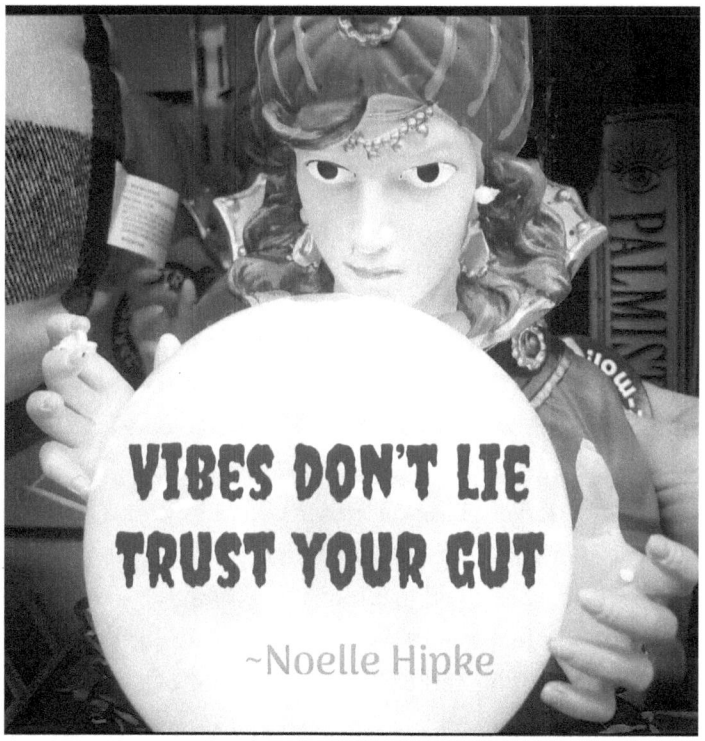

The friend I was planning to attend the yoga retreat with informed me they had gotten a used motor home for us to take.

I turned to her and said, "Did you get it from the city of Garden Grove?"

And she said "Yes. How did you know that?"

I shrugged, not realizing what was happening. She then let me know it was in the shop for repairs. And I said, "Is it going to be $1,500 dollars?"

She said, "Yes. How did you know that?"

Well, it turns out that as I was clearing my system of toxins and poisons and putting in good-healthy energy through nutrition, exercise, and taking care of myself, I developed the ability to read and sense other people's vibrational energy. They didn't have to say a word.

This tendency is why you feel good around some people and not so good around others. If an individual is bogged down with negativity and toxicity, they send you their signals. We can all be telepathic. All you have to do is clear, cleanse, and detoxify to activate your superpowers.

## SMELL

All of my senses amped up when I detoxified. My Spidey sense of smell was off the charts. My Human Design chart already shows I have extrasensory smell, but after detoxifying, I would ride my bike by someone who was six feet away and smell their cologne. I could smell cancer; it smells metallic.

I will never forget going on a date with a guy who ate a special diet. I knew something was off when I hugged him. He had a funky smell that repelled me. I had met him at a recent high school reunion. We went out and had a great first date, and I was attracted to him. We spent hours talking and connecting on a lot of topics. I enjoyed his company, but I couldn't get that smell out of my head. He walked me to the door and gave me a passionate kiss and then grabbed my boob. *What?* I said, "Did you just grab my boob?" He chuckled and thought that it was funny. Not sure what to make of it, I let it go but made a mental note.

A few days later, we talked on the phone after he got home from the gym late at night and made plans to see each other the next day. I invited him to pop in when I was on my lunch break at work. I just wanted to see if he still had that funky smell or if it was a one-time thing. When he arrived at my job, he gave me a hug, and I smelled that strong odor again. My higher self practically shouted at me, "NO. He is not the one for you." I spent a few minutes showing him around, and then he took off. I sat in silence to process how this information had come in so loud and clear from my senses alone.

The very next night, I was invited to go out for a girls' night. One of my friends happened to bring a girl from my high school who had attended the same recent high school reunion. When I saw her, I told her I had gone on a few dates with the guy from our recent reunion. She asked me how it went. Not wanting to divulge my true reasoning, I just said we were not a good match.

About ten minutes later, she approached me to tell me she had been dating that guy for months and had been with him the night he and I had spoken.

I said, "That's funny, 'cause he said he was at the gym working out when in actuality he was with you and then called me on his way home after your date." *Ding ding.* Another light bulb moment.

I looked at her and noticed how similar we looked—slim, long straight hair, blue eyes. And I said, "Let's take a picture of us together and send it to him."

So that is exactly what we did. I texted, "Gym, huh? Well, at least you have good taste. She looks a lot like me." And that was the end of it for me. On our very first date, I had told him I could be intuitive. Little did he know I was going to prove myself right a few days later.

I tell you this because you have the universe in you. You can tap into your superpowers by not drinking and not doing drugs, detoxifying the body, and eating nutritious foods. It's as simple as that. Add the modalities I am sharing with you here, and you will be the manifester of your own creations.

I have used my sense of smell on many occasions to weed out people who are not good for me. And you can too. We have something called pheromones, which enable us to determine if we are a good match with someone based on smell. Sometimes you are attracted, while other times you are repelled. Use your senses. They are your superpowers.

## BREATHWORK

My first experience with breathwork was at the free yoga retreat I won a ticket to. My friend and I drove the used motorhome down to Joshua Tree National Park, stalling at every light on the two-hour drive. However, the universe led us there safe and sound. I literally dived into the retreat upon arrival, ditching all my friends and focusing hard on my own healing journey.

I noticed a long line around one of the buildings and decided to investigate. It was for a breathwork session I had passed on the day before because of the title: Chop Wood and Carry Fire. It had sounded like a lot of work to me. But I decided to give it a try since I felt the urge to do so. The room was packed with hundreds of people side by side on their yoga mats, practically touching. They often have to turn away people due to max capacity.

I looked around the room and beheld all the beautiful auras. Many of us were half naked because we were in the desert and it was about 100 degrees out. Women and men of all ages radiated, and I mean *radiated*, superpower energies. These people were taking care of themselves, putting nutritional food in their bodies, not drinking, not partying, exercising, and doing the work on themselves. I could see it and I could sense it. I wanted what they had.

As we went into the breathing exercises, the energy in the room changed dramatically. We moved energy in the body, and the teacher led us through chants, songs, music, words, thoughts, energies, symbolism, animal totems, and the universe. It was a very powerful energetic exchange.

Shamanism has been around for centuries, and for very good reason—to keep us connected to our history, roots, ancestors, and each other. Healers, hippies, and Native American traditions are a few things that will help heal humans on this planet. They represent a future of freedom, health, happiness, peace, traditions, respect, and purity, for they have learned to live off the land, and materialism does not dictate their lifestyle. Native American belief systems have been around for centuries but were tossed aside and uprooted when European cultures took over. The new culture became consumed with trading, gold, farming, travel, technology, growth, consumerism, materialistic gain, control, developing, and taking over without giving much thought to humankind and Mother Nature.

During my breathing experience, I heard people yelling and crying as they released stuck energy in their bodies. It was surreal. My mind's eye opened up, and visions of the phoenix, pyramids, lotus flower, and chakra colors flooded my third eye. The woman next to me started crying loudly. Tears rolled down my own face as I released stuck emotions that had lain dormant—pain, misery, beauty, harmony, all back to back. The emotions and energy that flooded that room and the accompanying sounds created an experience I will never forget. It was a bit eerie at first, but once you learn and understand the transformation that is happening, you realize it needs to take place in order to heal the body and soul.

As the woman next to me cried, one of my favorite songs by Sarah McLachlan came on: "Angel." They had played this song at the funeral of my best friend, who had committed suicide. At that moment, I felt the urge to sing at the top of my lungs. Full disclosure: I am not a very good singer, but I felt compelled to send out love. As I sang, "In the arms of an angel" with my eyes closed and a scarf over my face, I saw an angel floating above me, and the crying woman next to me started to sing with me. She had come out of her transformation and gone into healing mode by releasing and accepting. I knew the angel was healing us.

Breathwork is incredible energy healing that most people will never understand unless they let go and give it a try.

I ended up doing one more breathwork session the next day, which led me to begin healing. My husband had left me a few weeks earlier, and it was like all the pieces of my heart were strewn across the floor, and I was picking them up one by one—twenty-six years of memories, events, lifetime achievements.

You see, my husband had moved out of the house when I was out of the country, in New Zealand. The crazy part was that while I was away, I found myself crying during yoga. An energy connection was being broken. I didn't understand why I was having these crazy emotions, but I had the urge to not go back home. When I did, the shoe dropped. I was surprised to see him at the airport in grungy clothes without the kids in tow. When we were getting off the freeway at our exit, he told me that he and my son had moved out. I walked into the house in a daze, noticing his things had been removed from the garage and closet. I was in complete shock. A sense of betrayal filled my body and soul. My five-year-old daughter was excited to see me after two weeks, but I was not present at all. I was numb and trying to figure out if this was a nightmare or reality.

That breathwork session helped heal part of my heart in an instant. I had a long way to go, but it was a good start. Nothing happens overnight when it comes to the body and soul healing. It takes time, lessons, and awareness.

During the rest of that retreat, I didn't shower for three days and used baby wipes to clean up and sunblock to protect my skin. I was in the midst of deciding if I should try to work out my marriage or move on and get a divorce.

My husband and I were going to counseling, and I sensed he was setting me up to be the bad mom because he did not want to work things out. His religious beliefs were different than mine, so he constantly belittled and badgered me about this. But when you are religious, aren't you supposed to embrace everyone? Love everyone unconditionally no matter what they believe? He told me, "You are into Buddhism, and that is not right." In reality, I embraced all religions. I was forced to become Catholic as a kid, and I was the one who brought our family to a Christian church.

No one has the right to inflict their religious beliefs on anyone. Ultimately, religion is what divided us. He believed people who didn't believe the Christian way and did believe in extrasensory perceptions were witches. However, the fact of the matter is that we all have extrasensory perceptions if we are tuned into them. He told me I was too sensitive. If there were no sensitive people, how do you think the world would be? He didn't understand superpowers, wasn't aligned, didn't know how to access his own, and never wanted to understand. He shut me down constantly, poking holes in my aura and energy field. And this went on for over a decade, tanking my health. I began to wonder if in a past life he'd burned women at the stake and had carried that over to this lifetime in his DNA. However, as he didn't believe in past lives, I am sure he would never consider this as an option.

During the day that followed the retreat, rhyming poetry—eleven typed pages' worth—flowed out of me as I transformed my mind, body, and soul and came into alignment. Breathwork offered me insight into what was happening around me over the years. I levitated above my home while in meditation, watching what felt like a movie. I saw myself and my family in the house, interacting, demonstrating the negative energies that had existed there for quite some time. He had been plotting, planning, and deceiving me for a while—preparing documents and noting anything he might be able to use in court against me.

We had a counseling session scheduled with the church counselor for that evening. I called the counselor and told her we needed to cancel our appointment and asked him to meet me for dinner instead. We had dinner, and after we ate, I read the poem out loud to him, calling him out on all the things he had done to me and everything we had experienced together. Remember, it was eleven pages typed, so I went on for a good ten minutes or so.

In the end I told him, "I set you free." I never again wanted anything to do with anybody who would treat and disrespect me this way. We are supposed to be beings of unconditional love, not judgments and deceit. I could tell he was shocked, bewildered, and I knew I was right on point. It was the ultimate callout, and nobody could have said it better than my higher self, who witnessed the entire movie play out.

Our higher selves see things, know things, and guide us to what is right for us. The incredible gift of wisdom, clarity, healing, and knowingness was granted to me through breathwork—which led me to become a breathwork guide a few years down the road. It was one of the best gifts of transformation, clarity, and healing a soul could accomplish.

Breathwork is now used in addiction, drug, and alcohol recovery centers.

## TIPS ABOUT SUPERPOWERS

- Certain aspects are more enhanced than others.
- Everybody has different superpowers.
- Respect each other's superpowers; honor your differences.
- You never know what is going on in someone else's life or head.
- Give people space to allow them to be themselves; accept them for who they are.
- Do not judge. Observe and learn.
- Do not be envious or jealous.
- Write down your superpowers so you can focus and enhance them.
- How do you stand when you want to activate your superpowers?
- What does your superpower feel like? Sound like?
- Exercise gets energy flowing, creating clarity, energy, high vibration.
- Music is frequency healing, happiness, high vibration.
- Write down your friends' superpowers.
- Activate your superpowers; ignite when needed.

## MOTHER NATURE: OUR GROUNDING FORCE

I talked about grounding earlier, but I'll go more in depth here. Mother Nature is the mother lode of healing for the earth and each other. Trees carry amazing wisdom from decades and decades of being rooted and withstanding weather changes, the environment, animals, humans, and planets. They are connected through their very own underground network of communication—like the internet. They carry healing forces and vibrational messages.

The five elements are earth, water, fire, air, and space/ether. I learned a lot about connecting to the earth when I dated a musician who was a creative earth sign. He taught me how important it was to ground to the earth. He took me on amazing trips to Big Sur, where we would just stand in awe, overlooking majestic nature scenes of the ocean and forest. The energy filled my body with pure enlightenment. We would take walks on the beach or just sit in the sand. We would go on hikes to a waterfall. It was romantic and healing all the way around. It was his way of life, and I'll forever be grateful that he got me to see, feel, understand, and witness.

From there, I took things a bit further and started taking my shoes off and walking on the earth barefoot. That is when I really learned and felt grounded to the earth. Walking in sand, grass, or dirt barefoot clears our bodies of negative energetic patterns and fills us up with healing ones. The soles of your feet are connected to every single organ in your body. When you remove your shoes, you energetically connect to the earth and each other on a cellular, vibrational, and magnetic level. It is one of the most healing things you can do every day for your body.

I often took my daughter to the largest park in our city; I preferred it over the beach because vibrational energy is higher among trees. Notice how you feel when you are outside in certain environments.

See how you resonate with the earth and how it resonates with you. Connect, release, receive, realign.

Go on picnics to heal the body with food and Mother Nature. It's a double whammy.

Water is also a natural vibrational healing force. Just as sound travels through water five times better than air, you reap the benefits of Mother Nature five-fold when you swim in the ocean, natural springs, lakes, etc. And do you remember all the properties I shared with you in the beginning of this book about living water? Your body will absorb all of this living, healing water. That is why surfers are so dang happy and chill.

## The Healing Field

As I mentioned earlier, I had a meltdown when the city chopped down our healing field of trees. I eventually learned to accept it and realized the tragedy might carry a message to uproot myself after twenty-four years in the same home.

My higher self told me to fill my house with lots of new plants to fill in the healing energy field around me and my daughter. So that is what I did. Mother Nature heals us. We are tree huggers because we can see, feel, and sense their energy and messages. People who disrespect nature and don't understand are often destructive to you, the environment, and themselves. We can plant new trees, but they will never carry the same vibrational wisdom messages or be as pure as the previous ones.

Those who set out to invade other people or territories are destroying all of us, which is why we can feel it even if we are on the other side of the earth. We are all connected as one, through energy. So if the news says something bad is happening, even if it isn't, our bodies may believe it and create it. That is how powerful human conscious energy really is. No religion, no nationality, no beliefs, no politics should separate us. We should all love and accept each other unconditionally. That is the secret of healing the planet, our souls, and each other.

Our bodies are some of the most intelligent life forces on the planet. We can use them for good or bad. Our bodies adapt, reject, and react to what is happening around us and within us. Honoring and respecting your soul and the souls of others creates peace.

Keys to soul healing:

- Compassion, forgiveness, and unconditional love toward everyone
- Health leads to happiness.
- Money can't buy self-love.
- Money can't buy health.
- You can't have wealth if you don't have health.

In case you need a reminder, here are the eight Rs to soul healing:

1. Retreat
2. Rest
3. Relax
4. Release
5. Repair
6. Recharge
7. Reset
8. Realign

Use your energy to build, not destroy, by committing to the following:

- Meditate
- Educate
- Create
- Generate

Good health starts within your body—mind, heart, gut, organs, blood, skin, hair, eyes, teeth, and cells.

What has changed your life for the better in this book? What little tweaks can you make to improve your life? A person stagnates if they're only focused on themselves. If we share our energy with the right people, we can do so much good for this planet.

You will use these tools for the rest of your life and pass them down to the next generations. You are amazing. You have the superpowers to change the world for the better. You are creating the new world order.

• • •

## SLEEP

Sleep is the fountain of youth. It helps heal the cells and regenerate the skin, organs, eyes, and bones—every single inch of your body inside and out. And when you are a blossoming teenager, you need more of it. Your body is growing in leaps and bounds.

Dreams allow you to astral travel and gain enlightenment, transcendence, and multiple perspectives from different dimensions of the soul, including the higher self. This data comes in the form of symbols, feelings, sensations, etc.

We spend one-third of our lives sleeping. Some advice to get the most out of your sleep:

- Make sure you have a good mattress.
- No electronics one hour before bedtime allows you to shut down the mind.
- The body needs time to adjust and shut down. Dim lights in the home in the evening.
- Use blue-light glasses to block the light from computers, phones, and devices.
- Stick to a set bedtime. The body likes a sleep routine.
- People who think they don't need a lot of sleep and don't sleep are not reaching their highest potential.

- The body processes daily information as it sleeps.
- You will gain needed info when you sleep even if you don't remember.
- Turn off your phones when you sleep and don't keep anything electronic running by your bedside.
- Your brain is recording the interaction and exchange of invisible information for you to access at a later date and time.
- Elevate to higher frequencies to get a new, clear perspective on how to do things better.
- Use an air purifier. This cleans the air, which enables your body to heal even faster when it is sleeping.
- Use a humidifier. This puts moisture in the air, which helps our lungs, eyes, and skin stay healthy and moist. This slows down aging and hydrates the body.

## ACUPUNCTURE

Acupuncture is another form of alternative medicine and a component of traditional Chinese medicine in which thin needles are inserted at the meridian points of the body. Pay attention to these ancient traditions. They have survived for good reason.

The practice of acupuncture started in China approximately 3,000 years ago. Acupuncture was long considered a pseudoscience in the West, which basically means it was discredited because there wasn't enough evidence of its efficacy. We have only recently developed the technology to track and prove the effects. What cracks me up is that people will believe in God, which is an invisible energy not backed by science, but they won't believe in other invisible energies that are not backed up by science.

It has taken forty years for acupuncture treatments to become accepted in the United States. More and more health insurance providers are covering this practice.

## DENTAL CARE

Dental care insurance doesn't cover much in the US besides X-rays, two teeth cleanings a year, and a bit of a discount on other services. I highly recommend you make the effort to get your teeth cleaned every six months. Do not ignore a toothache or a funky pain. Your body is trying to tell you something you will have to deal with sooner rather than later.

My friends who were practicing dentists moved from the US to New Zealand to open up a dental practice. They are very smart businesspeople. A few years back, the New Zealand healthcare system offered free dental work for children until the age of seventeen. I am not sure if they still cover the same today. However, most of the time, the parents waited until right before the kids turned seventeen to take them in. They were often hit hard with a lot of dental work all at once.

My friends figured out how to make the system work better. They worked with the schools and hired buses to bring kids into the dentist office, and they performed the work and sent the kids back to school. All the parents had to do was sign a waiver.

You really need to pay attention to your teeth. They are connected to all the organs in your body, your chakras, your meridians—everything. Ever notice how many elderly people have dentures? There really should be a better option. Implants are a good solution, but be prepared to spend $3,000 and upwards to get one tooth done. That adds up really quickly when insurance doesn't cover much.

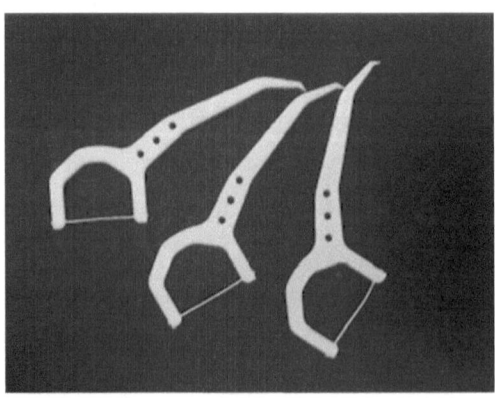

Brush your teeth every morning and every night. And don't forget to floss *first*, before you brush. Use those easy-to-maneuver floss toothpicks from the dollar store.

## MINDSET

Remember, our minds have the power to create anything—even if we don't want them to. Taking the time to program your mind is a key component to living a happy and healthy life.

I heard stories on three different occasions where people who were scheduled to get COVID tested in 2020 decided not to go to their appointment due to no illness symptoms, and all three a few days later received a letter in the mail stating they had COVID. Something is beyond fishy here. I have a feeling a lot of people who got COVID out there did it to themselves, by convincing the cells in their body they had something they did not.

We become what we think and believe to be true. When faced with any situation that challenges you, reprogram your mind, and you can realign with your true self.

## WATER: FLOW FLUSHING

Living water cleanses the mind, body, and soul. So it is important to get the highest quality water you can afford to flush out your system and keep your organs clean. Living water offers organisms to keep you thriving over surviving; there is a big difference. Hydration is key. Which is exactly why I put it as the very first chapter in this book. This is a substance we put into our bodies our entire lives and which offers us one of the highest possible vibrations when used correctly in conjunction with nutrition.

Bottled water wastes many containers, and the plastic from the bottles is not good for you or the environment. I had been buying bottled pH water with electrolytes before I installed the home water filtration system. When Spring Aqua was installed in my home, I got my own special faucet with a pH balance of 7.5 on the left and 9.5 on the right. I started using the 7.5 pH water to wash and soak all my fruits and veggies, my teas, my oatmeal. Heck, I didn't even realize how much water I used. I became very grateful for my healing water—especially when I noticed a large difference in my house plants after I watered them with the special water. They blossomed, grew new leaves, radiated, and their energy became high vibration. When I saw how much they were elevating their frequency, I realized I must be doing the same. Healing begins from the inside.

You can learn more about this topic at https://www.LuminaryHealingCenter.com.

## PEMF: PULSATED ELECTROMAGNETIC FIELD THERAPY

To reiterate, my life changed for the better when I discovered PEMF therapy. These mats send a low intensity pulsed electromagnetic field into the body in order to safely stimulate healthy muscles, which can temporarily increase microcirculation by up to 30 percent. The particular PEMF mat I utilize has a unique signal configuration that is patented, so not all mats are the same. It basically comes down to frequency.

PEMF mats enhance the following:

- Well-being
- Sleep
- Stress recovery
- Relaxation
- Energy
- Nutrients
- Oxygen
- Blood flow

- Waste removal
- Muscle conditioning
- Athletic performance
- Muscle recovery
- Physical fitness and strength

I enrolled in a local healing center to try out PEMF therapy. A cute elderly couple ran the center. They were in their seventies and skipping around like they were teenagers. They swore by this product. The husband would use PEMF therapy in the morning and then go on a mountain-bike ride. Who does that in their seventies? They were avid believers. My first session was free, and I bought a month unlimited option and booked my session for every day they were open, Monday through Friday, at 4 p.m.

After a month of receiving PEMF sessions, I decided to buy the system. This way I could use it whenever I wanted and take it with me when I traveled, not to mention share it with my kiddo. It was a bigger price tag than I wanted to pay, but I was desperate to get my health back. When you make good money working under a stressful environment, there is a good chance you will be using that good money to do anything to regain your health.

I have worked with senior citizens much of my life, and they would benefit greatly from PEMF therapy. Blood flow slows down and arteries close up as we age. Many seniors are not eating enough, have poor nutrition, and are dehydrated. The organs, eyes, skin, brain, etc., all suffer. PEMF mats help with getting nutrients into the system while triggering waste removal and speeding up blood flow for optimum health.

These mats should be everywhere, in every household. These mats have been linked to relief from PTSD, anxiety, depression, sleep deprivation, ADHD, pain, aches, stress, and the list goes on. Professional athletes use these devices to speed recovery between games. It is a miracle worker that has not really been brought to the forefront.

This technology will enable our bodies to thrive.

You have the power to own your health. You can work with anyone in the world. No one doctor is going to know how to treat all of you. You need multiple specialists to guide you, not to mention coaches, mentors, and trailblazers; and most of all, you need to listen to your higher self.

You can learn more about this topic and request a one-on-one consultation at https://www.LuminaryHealingCenter.com.

## FACIAL INJECTIONS

Did you know there is a 73.33 percent markup on Botox per unit? So, say it is $10 a unit; then they are making $7.33 per unit. That is damn good money.

I am going to be totally transparent here: I have done Botox in the past. I started out with twenty-two units and eventually went up to thirty. One time, I went to a new business and was told I would need sixty units of Botox. It would have cost me $600, and their profit would have been $440. From that point on, I had it in my head that I needed sixty units or more to keep up with it.

Check out these numbers, ladies. You have been bombarded with ads about how you need to look younger to have value. To do so, you are going to need to get these injections, have surgery, and spend lots of money. Talk about giving you a complex. "Here, let us douse you with toxic injections to make you feel good about yourself. And yes, we are going to inject it right by your brain and eyes." And really, no side effects?

We can come up with a holistic and healthy alternative. I have been researching that too. I want to show the world that we have the option to not age. The secret is eating healthy, living water, sleeping, exercising, relaxing, avoiding stress, nurturing yourself. And this is exactly what the younger generations are going to wake up and do. You are going to take better care of yourselves, be aware, listen to your higher selves, and make your own decisions. You will be independent, and it will be accepted and approved. You will live by your own standards—not what someone else wants of you.

## THE SWAN

Back in 2004, the reality television series *The Swan* hit America. The plastic surgery movement was projecting perfection and anti-aging. Women who felt they were "ugly ducklings" applied to get complete body makeovers. Perfection, fake, and over-the-top features were promised. These women got breast augmentations, tummy tucks, liposuction, upper arm tucks, Lasik eye surgery, complete dental makeovers, hair extensions, etc. You name it, they did it. And they did all these procedures at once or back-to-back in order to fit the show's timeline.

It is shocking to the central nervous system to undergo this type of process, let alone what is does to the body, mind, and soul. I remember watching in amazement at the age of thirty-four, somewhat horrified at what these women had undergone in order to make themselves feel better. The recovery consisted of changing their diet and exercising as well as psychological sessions, often revealing mental issues generated by being conditioned to believe they weren't pretty enough or average. Had they taken these steps in the first place, they may not have felt the need to take such drastic measures.

Aging naturally in the past was simply the way of life. I see the era of *The Swan* as a turning point in history, where plastic surgery took main stage, and the messages conveyed by its proponents programmed people everywhere to feel they had to look younger and prettier in order to be accepted by society.

## MICROCHANNELING

Microchanneling is the new alternative to microneedling, injections, and surgery. It is a holistic alternative that can be performed on any part of the body and is less damaging to the skin than microneedling. Microchanneling is a needle-stamping technique, whereas in microneedling, a needle is dragged across the skin. Microchanneling uses your natural healing powers to reshape the skin and texture.

And if you add in all the other extras I have shared with you in this book, your body will radiate good health from within. There are even nutritional supplements called "Botox in a bottle." Potent herb-based supplements can give you the healing powers you need to have stunning skin qualities. The healing modalities on aging holistically and looking fabulous will surface a lot more over the next few years. I find holistic health is the best way to slow down aging on all levels.

You can learn more about this topic at https://www.LuminaryHealingCenter.com.

## GROW YOUR OWN GARDEN

Another tip is to grow your own amazing healing garden. When I went to New Zealand, I noticed that everyone grew fruits and veggies in their gardens and brought them in to eat with their meals on a daily basis. We should all be doing that. You can grow a garden on your balcony. There are inventions enabling you to do so. We put our own love and energy into the plant as we water it, nurture it, and encourage it to grow. Think how amazing and excited we feel when we notice a large growth or change occurring in a plant. And then that amazing plant is consumed by our bodies. Voilà: pure magic love and nutrients entering our system. It's a direct upgrade.

Growing your own garden is empowering, fun, creative, nurturing, and magnificent.

• • •

## NATURAL NAILS, HAIR, AND SKIN

### Nails

In the 1990s I went to school to become a manicurist. Little did I know I would soon be phased out due to lower-priced nail places popping up everywhere. However, all skills and traits I have learned in my lifetime have benefited me in some way or another.

The only time I ever got acrylic nails was when I went to prom my junior year in high school. I got them the day of the event, and it was a nightmare. They were hot-pink with black flames to match my dress and looked pretty dang cool. But when I went to get ready for the big event, it turned into a disaster. I couldn't do a darn thing. I couldn't put on my earrings, I couldn't put on my makeup, and I couldn't do anything without fumbling all over the place. It was a total handicap. I had to be careful wiping my butt; I could claw my crotch if I wasn't careful. Those acrylic nails were weapons being used against me. I was helpless and hopeless. Within twenty-four hours, I ripped those suckers off and never looked back.

I have gone to doctors' offices and witnessed the young women who work there wearing pointy, colorful nails. Let me tell you, ladies: these often don't look pretty past the first day you put them on. Do you know how much bacteria are under those nails? And you are working in a doctor's office? To me, this signals a dirty environment. And you can't type worth a damn; I know that from experience. Your actions are limited when you have these nails on, and they are expensive. I would say I have easily saved $30,000 in my lifetime by doing my own nails. Now, that is a lot of money for something you have nothing to show for in the end. Can't you smell all those chemicals when you walk into the salon? You are putting that right onto your body, breathing it in, and the beat goes on.

What is in style is natural nails. You can get your natural nails to grow if you eat right, don't bite them, buff them, and keep nail polish on them. That's all you have to do.

## Hair

What does healthy, thick, shiny hair say? It says you eat well, you are healthy, you take care of yourself, and you have good DNA.

I highlighted my hair for many decades. I barely saw my natural hair color past the age of twelve. It damaged my hair, removed shine, and caused split ends. In my fifties, I realized true beauty lies in the natural color of my hair, given to me when I was born. When I grew my natural hair out in my fifties, it had a shine and sheen that it never had before. Why? Because I was eating better, taking supplements, drinking better water, sleeping more, and taking better care of myself.

After I turned fifty, I became concerned a man wouldn't want me if I didn't look ten years younger; after all, that is what society teaches us. Then I decided I didn't want a man in my life who would prioritize looks over mental connection and stimulation. Still, at one point I became very fearful of aging, which in turn brought on more aging—a process many women go through when they hit the big five-oh. I have surrendered to this and have realized that I am here to show you the beauty you can radiate from the inside out when you accept yourself, love yourself, and become the highest version of yourself. The right one will find you at the right time.

All your body parts were designed to enhance and radiate your true soul essence. We end up masking it and altering it based on what society tells us we should be doing: coloring our hair, tanning our bodies, putting on nails. It's a total joke. It can be fun for a while, but eventually you will realize that your natural beauty far outweighs all those so-called enhancements. By the way, PEMF sessions and nutrition help with healthy hair growth, too. I should know; my eyelashes are glorious!

## Skin

Skin care should always be a priority. I got a book on Korean skin care recommended by the *Dr. Phil* show when I was in my mid-forties. It had a lot of good recommendations for protecting your skin and what products to use. Korean women stay out of the sun, covering themselves with umbrellas, gloves, and long sleeves and pants. They do this to save the beauty of their skin. Again, by learning from what other cultures are doing, we can incorporate their healthiest practices into our lives. I started purchasing their recommended products from Amazon, and my skin changed for the better within six months. I am sure it also helped that I gave up red meat and changed my nutrition, but the combination of the two made all the difference in the world.

I have lived by the beach most of my life, so tanning was a way of life that I thought reflected healthy living. However, tanning will ruin your skin. It causes accelerated aging you don't see until you are much older. Sure, you might have a golden tan in your twenties. But that glow pales in comparison to the results that show up years later. Women who spend a lot of time in the sun, particularly if their country is close to the equator, show signs of aging at a much younger age. In order to look better in your golden years, take precautions in your earlier years.

Something that my mother never did for me that I did for my daughter was instill the habit of putting on sunblock at a young age. This will prevent some of those wrinkles. Use sun protection at all times. Stay out of the sun during the peak hours of 11 a.m. to 4 p.m.

If you are going to be outside, wear a hat to protect your face and eyes, and always wear sunglasses. Sunglasses helps prevent crow's feet that come from squinting all the time. And they protect your eyes. The sun is a powerful star that generates energy we need for our bodies, such as vitamin D, but overdoing it is not good for you.

Avoid tanning beds. I will never forget. I worked at a tanning bed salon and always seemed to burn the skin on my chest. I remember going to my Asian doctor in my early twenties and him saying that the skin on our chests is very thin. You don't want to burn it, because it will show your age. A lot of us are only concerned about our faces. But we need to consider our entire bodies. Make sure you spend the extra bucks on a really good sunscreen. After seeing a dermatologist, I discovered that most of the brands we get at Target and other grocery locations don't have UVA and UVB ray blocking. You will probably spend upwards of $40 for a decent sunblock that truly protects your skin from UVA and UVB rays; double-check that it protects against both. You will also need to reapply the sunblock every ninety minutes, so plan to take it with you when you head out, and don't leave it in the heat of the car.

As for self-tanning lotions, those products are toxic. And when you put the product on your skin, the toxins go right into your body and bloodstream. You smell funky, too. Isn't that a sign it might not be good for you? If you are light skinned, you are meant to be light skinned. Honor your genes and allow them to shine through.

In my early fifties, I noticed a woman close to my age with the most amazing, creamy, flawless white skin I had ever seen on a woman her age.

I said to her, "Your skin looks so pretty."

She said, "Oh no, I am so white. I have been trying to sit in the sun to get some color."

I said, "No, don't. You will ruin your skin. Keep it just the way it is. Your true beauty is radiating out. You are meant to be that color."

So, what I want you to take away here is the importance of doing your homework and creating good habits that protect you to the best of your abilities. Wear sunglasses (you will get so used to wearing them that you eventually won't be able to go outside without them), wear hats, wear sunblock, cover your arms and legs when you ride your bike or are going to be outside for long periods of time. Work in the garden early in the morning or later in the day when the sun levels aren't as strong.

I've learned that the sun sends us coded messages through its rays. When you go outside and spend time in the sun, consider the thoughts and feelings that come to mind. Spending time in the sun boosts our mood thanks to the vitamin D, opening you up to other realms. Think luminary rays of light hitting your body, healing you, guiding you. It really is magic. All of these precautions are important because you *must* spend some time outside in the sun in order to reap the benefits and power up your superpowers.

· · ·

## THINK DIRTY APP

I want to share an app called Think Dirty. This app allows you to scan items at the store to see how toxic they are for your body. I use it to scan lotions, shampoos, body washes, and deodorants. The app ranks the product on a scale from one to ten. The higher the number, the worse it is for the body. I tend to focus on getting as close to five on the scale as I can, meaning something is half as toxic as the products hitting the top of the charts. The app gives you a breakdown of the ingredients in the products and warns you of the chemicals.

I heard about this app when listening to an Australian podcast years ago. This is why I recommend watching and listening to what other countries are doing. Tune in, and you will gather insights on your own.

• • •

## REFLEXOLOGY

I learned about reflexology when I went to school to become a manicurist. Reflexology is an alternative medical practice that involves the application of pressure to specific points in the feet and/or hands. You can look up reflexology online and check out the diagrams on hands and feet to see which parts of the body are attached to each organ. It is rather remarkable. Reflexology helps alleviate stress and gives relief and relaxation.

### Foot Fetish

In my mid-forties, while going through a divorce, I decided to try something that didn't turn out like I expected. If someone asked me to name my favorite body part on me, I would have to say my feet. I have been blessed with beautiful feet, thanks to my DNA. My friends and men have complimented me on my feet. I have to say it is a pretty good asset to have because I see them a lot. Thank you, feet.

So, one day I was looking for a way to bring in some creative income and remembered that some people have fetishes involving feet. I decided to attend a foot-fetish party—basically an event where men pay you money so they can play with your feet. I enrolled to be a model online, sent in some photos of my feet, and was accepted as a model to line up with women half my age. I was okay with that because it was just my feet. Or so I thought.

My girlfriend and I drove up to Los Angeles where this private party was taking place. I didn't have the nerve to go in sober, and I was still drinking at the time, so we pounded a few beers in the car before we entered. Upon entering a dark room, I noticed a DJ in the corner, an open dance floor, and private rooms off to the side. They had asked us to dress in a school-girl theme, which wasn't an issue for me since I went to private school and had worn the uniform, so I knew what they expected. I wore my cute Michael Kors sandals to show off my freshly painted toenails.

We hadn't even been in the door two minutes when someone asked me to step aside and go into a room.

I said, "We just got here; let me feel things out, and I will circle back to you."

A beautiful girl from another local county came over to greet us. She directed us to a room where a photographer would be taking photos. I grabbed the photographer's attention across the room, and he came over to talk to me. I told him I did not want my face photographed at all because I worked in a high-profile job (Realtor to the senior citizens) and didn't want to be recognized.

Well, the man was not happy with my request and refused to photograph my feet if I wouldn't let him photograph my face. So I decided not to take him up on the opportunity. Instead, my girlfriend and I danced to warm up to the environment. I tried to feel the energy and wrap my head around where we were, what was taking place, and how I was feeling. When I looked around at the private rooms, I could see people's legs and feet because the rooms were sectioned off by hanging curtains that didn't go all the way to the ground. There was a massage table in each room that the foot girl would lie down on.

After two songs, another man approached me for a private session. All of a sudden, I looked down at my feet, and it hit me like a bolt of lightning. My higher self told me, "You can't let these men touch your feet. These feet connect to your soul. That is why they are called the soles of your feet. When you let these men touch your feet, you are letting them touch your soul."

I would be letting a random man with shady energy right into my energy field, affecting my entire soul. You see, as I mentioned with regard to grounding, the soles of your feet are connected to every single organ and part of your body. What I thought was a harmless appendage to expose turns out to be one of the most intimate parts of my body. Maybe this is why these men have such a fetish with feet. They want to tap into soul energy.

Upon realization and immediate enlightenment, I turned to my girlfriend and said, "We gotta go." I was buzzed, but the guidance was loud and clear. I heard it and I followed it.

We ended up sitting in the car until the buzz wore off a bit and then drove right back home to Orange County. I wanted to go home and shuck off the energy I had been surrounded by. You see, these types of environments bring out dark energies and energy vampires—toxic people who are looking for someone they can suck the life force out of. Paying close attention to the energy in a room and how you feel and assessing the tone of a situation really helps you take a perspective you didn't see before.

· · ·

## ESSENTIAL OILS

Egyptians used oils in cosmetics and ointments as early as 4500 BC. Their herbal medicines and perfumes contained myrrh, cedar, and grapes. Plants and herbs are power extracts that have been treasured as beauty-enhancing remedies and are often the base of today's pharmaceuticals. The Egyptians were known for their youthful appearance. Cleopatra's legendary beauty is believed to have been due to her use of Egyptian clays, Dead Sea salts, essential oils, and fatty oils.

Other cultures that have used extracts for beauty care include India, China, Rome, and Greece. The Greek physician Hippocrates shared medicinal uses for over 300 plants with the medical community. He believed diffusing aromatics in the city of Athens to combat the plague, a process they called fumigation, was beneficial. He spoke about how essential oils, diffused or applied, can affect the internal organs and tissues of the body. Now do you see why Mother Nature is so important? She offers amazing healing qualities in the plants we consume, wear, and connect with.

Essential oils are part of the Indian Ayurvedic healthcare system. Historically, Indian doctors have offered ginger, myrrh, cinnamon, coriander, and sandalwood oils to their patients. Ayurvedic health is a natural healing system blending spiritual, philosophical, and practical elements. It has been practiced for at least 5,000 years and is still widely practiced in India today.

## Essential Oils of Today

I purchased a set of oils in 2010 before my daughter came into the world. I wanted an alternative to heal her holistically should the need arise. I used lavender nightly on her when she was a baby and still do to this day. I put it on her feet so it goes directly into her organs, offering a calming effect. I put in on my feet, wrists, neck, and behind my ears, and inhale the scent before going to sleep.

Over the years, I have purchased many different brands. I diffuse them and refer to them when we have health issues: ear aches, sore throats, moods/feelings, want elevation, etc. I have a book I use to look up health issues, and it guides me on how to work the oil into the body for the best holistic healing benefits. I use oils on my breathwork clients in order to activate the chakras and move energy through the body. Oils amplify the process by setting in motion the cells in our body to energize, revitalize, and release.

When I'm working on this book, I put on oils to elevate and expand my mind. Special oil blends can be placed on your third eye for activation or the top of your head to move up into the transcendence and ascension state.

Essential oils have been around for a very long time and have circulated in many cultures. And they've gained popularity for a reason: they work. I have purchased many off the beaten path, from other countries and cultures. I provide essential oil company recommendations on my website.

• • •

## HYPNOSIS

Hypnosis became a popular treatment for medical conditions in the late 1700s when effective pharmaceutical and surgical treatment options were limited. It was originally used to induce dreams, which were analyzed to get to the root of the trouble.

I have worked with hypnosis healers on several occasions. I believe it would be beneficial if more therapists brought this technique into their daily practice with patients. It opens gateways to our subconscious and unconscious minds, which allows us to process and understand ourselves on multiple levels. Think upgrade. I've ended up with three pages of typed notes at the end of some sessions. The insights, visions, and messages are truly remarkable and revolutionary to self-health.

This technique is best utilized when working with an established professional in their field. Even though this technique has been around the block, pioneering techniques by modern psychologists, physicians, and researchers are taking it to the next level.

## NEURO-LINGUISTIC PROGRAMMING (NLP)

Neuro-linguistic programming has been used by coaches, therapists, and healers for many years. NLP picks up and alters an individual's subjective vision of the world. NLP is not hypnotherapy. It functions through the conscious mind by using language to bring about changes in thoughts and behaviors. That is why affirmations and listening and saying things as you move the body helps reprogram the brain.

NLP is a psychological approach that connects language, patterns of behavior, and thoughts learned through specific outcomes and experiences.

By asking questions and writing down the things you would like to change in your life, you self-evaluate and bring in NLP to create a new brain pattern and result. By reframing your belief system, you can apply new meanings to certain behaviors, thereby enabling you to believe in, imagine, and create the world you want.

## EMOTIONAL FREEDOM TECHNIQUE (EFT), I.E., TAPPING

I have been using the emotional freedom technique since 2010 when I had one of the most traumatic experience of my life. (I intend to write more about this topic at a later date, in another book.) To help me move forward, a practitioner tapped on a series of meridian points on my body. When you tap in a certain order, stating a series of words, you can open up the energy patterns and repattern them. You tap on the hands, the head, the chest, the face, and continue in a certain order repeatedly to set the program into place. Not very many people knew about this technique in 2010, but over the years it has gotten recognition and become more mainstream.

EFT/tapping is a great way to get an immediate release of pent-up energy and can be easily learned to perform on yourself or others. I believe in the beginning I paid around $250 for the session because it was not a well-known technique. Getting certified in some of these holistic healing modalities is rather expensive, time consuming, and exhausting, so that is often reflected in the price. Today there is an app you can pay for on your phone that will give you daily techniques and new teachings to incorporate into your life on a daily basis. Now, that is pretty amazing.

## AYAHUASCA/PSYCHEDELICS

Ayahuasca has long been used as a medicine by the people of the Amazon basin. It is basically a brew made with plants that put people into an altered state of mind, causing hallucinations. I have considered undertaking an ayahuasca journey. I even put down a deposit but never attended. I was told by another healer that if you are in a good state of mind, you should not attempt this.

However, from friends and healers, I hear ayahuasca has profound benefits and helps people overcome blockages in their lives. And this may very well be the best route now and in the future for therapists working with psychiatric patients in order to fast-track right to the problem. This drug has been utilized by psychologists to help clear and realign a patient's subconscious programming.

What you need to know about this drug-induced mental clearing is that you get very sick to the point of throwing up and then enter a transcendent state. You will see things in other dimensions and be taken into other realms to understand the complicated unknown. If you choose to go on this type of journey, you will need the proper guide.

## TIMELINE HEALING

Timeline healing is a comprehensive method that leads to quantum psychic healing on all levels of existence: physical, emotional, mental, astral, ethereal, causal, spiritual,—universal basically moving between the holographic fields of space, time, and dimensions. Expect your energy to be vacillating through the body, breath, mind, intellect, memory, ego, soul/self. It's a form of interdimensional soul-travel healing. Timeline healing is a tool for dealing with problems that are unknown to us, originating from early childhood or previous lives. You become aware of your past lives while actively healing your specific past self, which in turn is reflected in your present self. In essence, this method uses energy to connect your past, present, and future self to create the timeline you want to achieve. This type of healing can create genetic healing of ancestors and of ancestral fingerprints found inside you and is a monumental healing tool.

## REIKI

Reiki is a Japanese energy healing technique that promotes relaxation and reduces stress and anxiety. Since our bodies are made up of energy, the Reiki practitioner works with your energy field, manipulating it with their hands to improve the flow and balance in your body to support healing. This type of healing can be offered by touching or not touching the body.

Reiki comes from two Japanese words: "Rei," which means universal, and "ki," which translates to a life force energy. Reiki has been around since the 1920s, over 100 years. It is newer compared to some of the other healing modalities mentioned. However, since I cover force field and biofield in this book, it should be acknowledged.

## MASSAGE THERAPY

Massage is the manipulation of the body's soft tissues using hands, fingers, elbows, knees, forearms, feet, or a device. Massage reduces pain, spasms, and nerve compression; offers relaxation by lowering heart rate, respiratory rate, and blood pressure; and boosts the immune system and decreases stress.

I have been receiving massage therapy healing for many years and find it to be very beneficial whether I am married or single. As a single woman I've joked that I have to pay someone to touch me, but I look forward to the massage therapist using his healing hands on me. When getting a message, pay attention to how you feel, your surroundings, and how the therapist makes you feel. Some therapists have better healing capabilities than others. Some push too hard, while others make me tingle, relax, and center. Each healer is going to offer something different, and on some days, one will feel better than another. Why? Because their energy is affected by the clients they work on. Remember, energy is transferred, so make sure you work with someone who is intentional, directional, and professional and has taken the time to clear their own energy.

There are many types of massages offered at spas all over the world: Swedish, hot stone, aromatherapy, deep tissue, sports, trigger point, reflexology, shiatsu, Thai, prenatal, couple, chair, lymphatic, cranial sacral (head), and abhyanga oil (Ayurveda), to name a few.

## SAGING/SMUDGING

Saging is a traditional technique of smoke cleansing that has its roots in the Native American tradition of smudging. The process stems from the idea that energy is all around us and within everything. To sage/smudge, dried sage leaves are burned, and the smoke removes negative energy, cleansing and purifying the space or person. The benefits to saging include purifying, symptom relief, release of negativity, cleansing or charging objects, mood boosting, stress relief, elevated sleep quality, brain boosting, energy boosting, and aromatherapy.

We are borrowing from another culture here to bring in this healing modality. My Native American friend talks about saging when we want to shift the energy around us and in our homes. She often gifts sage to me, emphasizing the extra power infused into it when it is given by a Native American.

There were times as a Realtor that it was difficult for me to sell a house because the homeowner's energy was so strong in it. They may have lived there for many years or died in the home, which many cultures feel is taboo. On one occasion, I had a hard time getting offers on a great home that had been completely remodeled. I asked the homeowners to take down all their family photos in order to remove their energy and asked them to leave so I could smudge the home before the next open house. They were very religious, so I didn't know how well this idea would go over; however, for centuries many churches have used incense to clear energy. The smoke of incense is symbolic of purification. The homeowners allowed me to sage their home, and after the open house, we received several offers.

There is a lot of power and influence in energy.

My daughter attends after-school care, and there were days I could tell she was spun out from overload and energies from the other kids. She was absorbing negative energy and bringing it into our home. Some days, she didn't even look or act like herself. This didn't happen very often, but when it did, I brought out the sage. The moment I lit the sage and doused her with its intoxicating fumes, she would calm down. At points when we were struggling, we would do it every night before we went to bed. Then it tapered out as we moved through the stressful period. Still to this day, I will walk in to find her, at eleven years old, with sage in her hand, moving around the home. She seems to use it automatically when she feels the need. On this particular day, a tenant was moving out of part of our home. It was like she just knew it was time to clear our area.

Other types of energy-clearing herbs include the following:

- Cedar: a medicine of protection
- Palo santo: clears energy fields and connects to ancestors
- Wheatgrass: purifies and cleanses air

You can find these products online, along with other energy-cleansing processes.

## FENG SHUI

The philosophy of the Chinese practice of feng shui is that living spaces should be arranged to create balance with the natural world. The goal is to harness energy forces and establish harmony between an individual and their environment. Remember, everything is energy. By finding the flow and working with it, you can use it to your advantage.

Sometimes when I listed home property for sale, I would ask the owner if I could move the furniture around. The way they had it arranged often didn't flow for me. I would make a few tweaks, rearrange the furniture, and add a plant or two, and the homeowners immediately felt a difference. And that was before I knew about feng shui! I was just following the energy flow as I personally felt it. In time, I was introduced to feng shui and learned the basics. This propelled me to learn about the Chinese New Year and their customs. Fascinated by these tried-and-true traditions, I acquired books, studied their practices, and implemented the ones that I thought were beneficial in my home.

In order to get the most benefit out of feng shui, I recommend hiring a professional practitioner to come into your home and business to work with the energy to create the optimum success foundation for you personally. Keep in mind they will need to come in from time to time to shift the energy as years and energies change. But it is well worth the investment when you harvest the benefits.

## FUTURE OF HEALING

What lies in the future of healing? Cutting edge technology channeled in from Extraterrestrials to humans. Believe it or not, humans are currently working together in unison with Extraterrestrials to heal the universe and one another. The energy around the earth is shifting to higher frequencies, while moving faster as the vail is thinning. As the vail thins and you vibrate higher, you will be able to see and understand new realities you did not see there before. Multiple perceptions and new types of species will be felt, seen and experienced on a deeper level. Think sensational multidimensional! Be prepared to expand and get glimpses of instant knowledge like a flash of lightening. Ascension is the time of changing your belief systems, programming and behavior patterns. Give yourself permission to relax, adjust and comprehend. You are altering your DNA, which requires many changes and adjustments to frequency. There will be times when you are recalibrating and will not quite feel like yourself anymore. Good news! You are moving into a better version of your new self.

Be on the lookout for new technologies to surface, such as energy spas, med beds, awakening devices, well-being protectors, conscious bio-current devices, synergistic signals, cranial vibrational devices, meditation amplifiers, energetic space purifiers, recorded signals, circulating electrons, information-radiating plates, cosmic memory, atmospheric solar projections, meteoritic iron facilitators, electromagnetic wave disruptors, vibrational acoustic therapy, energy and light therapy, consciousness-grounding devices, prayer and mantra projectors, quantum therapy, scalar technology, vortex chambers, rejuvenation technology, energy tools, coherence enhancers, vortex pulsing electromagnetic field therapy (VPEMF), enhanced health transformation centers, aura photography, bio-plasmic energy readers, vitality rays, cell-growth stimulators, reproduction sciences, crystal healing technology, frequency healing, vortex-based mathematics, energy enhancements, mathematic energy expression, quantum vortex generators, and a slew of new other products that are actually excellent for you and your body, enabling you to shift into a super-conscious state and helping you tap into your superpowers, moving toward ascension!

• • •

## IN CONCLUSION

The future of a healing harmony of heaven on earth includes the alchemy of the five transformational elements of aether, water, air, fire, and earth. Merging art, science, and spirituality quantum wave mechanics is the front line of the new earth.

Healing is all about focusing on lifting your vibration to the highest frequency possible using consciousness and mindset. When you do the work and get into alignment, you are powered up and amplifying your superpowers. I have given you a lot to think about and consider by looking at multiple cultures, bringing in all types of holistic healing modalities as well as knowledge from the aethers, and using futuristic nontraditional approaches such as mathematics, frequency, light, sound, vibration, crystals, signals, devices, herbs, oils, energy, organization, systems, boundaries, arrangements, etc. Don't forget the importance of water, detoxification, and nutrition. I devoted the beginning chapters of this book to those particular topics for a reason. These are the true components to a holistic healthy lifestyle.

## JOURNAL: Chapter 9

1. Which healing techniques do you currently use?
2. Which new healing techniques would you like to add to your life?
3. Research any healing techniques you would like to learn more about and take notes; add them to your journal for future reference.
4. What are your best "magic moment" memories? (Refer back to this when you are feeling down.)
5. What can you do to reprogram your brain for the better?
6. What types of daily frequency healing can you implement in your life?

   Gratitude Journal: I hope you are getting into the habit of being thankful for all your blessings. Continue to write down what you are grateful for each day.

## SNAPSHOT REVIEW

Take a photo of this list or write it down in your journal and put it up somewhere you can see it daily.

1. Water
2. Detox
3. Nutrition
4. Sleep
5. Exercise
6. Nature
7. Ditch devices
8. Read books
9. Podcasts, audiobooks
10. Music/frequency healing

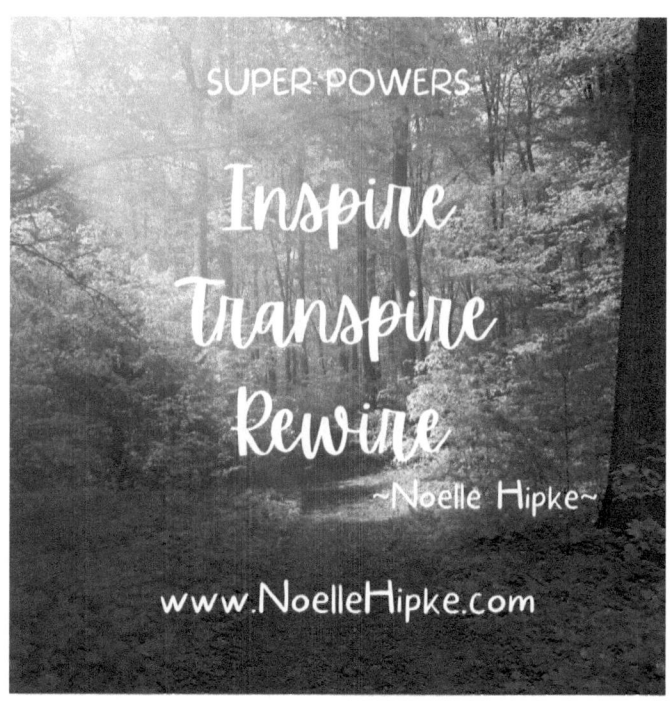

# CHAPTER 10

# SOUL HEALING

This chapter is going to open you up to a whole new world of professions and opportunities that have been kept on the down-low for the most part. The following professionals are trailblazers who have status, education, and are thinking outside the box. They don't so much follow traditional belief systems as they follow their instincts, hunches, self-guidance, and personal compass. They are innovators spearheading new trends toward understanding, comprehending, evaluating, manipulating, gauging, and analysis.

## LIGHTWORKERS AND LUMINARIES

Lightworkers, also known as luminaries, receive messages through light, sound, vibration, and telepathy to bring you new-earth healing techniques. Many of these healers are researchers and highly educated people thinking outside the norm. Lightworkers shake things up and wake up the beings that populate this amazing planet, linking them with their true divine spirit. The goal is to teach and model conscious expansion toward oneness and close the separation gap that occurs when people forget that they are a soul of light having a physical experience.

Lightworkers are divinely guided teachers and healers. They come in all different forms so that the right messages get delivered to the right people. I have stated as much throughout this book. I am being divinely guided to share wisdom and insights with you from all the knowledge I have acquired and received in this lifetime and—I believe—previous lifetimes.

Life has been a healing journey for me from the get-go. My years have been marked by loss, sadness, illness, depression, anxiety, loneliness, and fear so I could live through the storms and teach you how to use your internal compass. During turbulent periods, I have reinvented myself several times over in order to be the role model of living proof. Every single moment in my life has played a pivotal part in getting me to this point today.

Tips about lightworkers and luminaries:

1. Lightworkers are open to feeling other energetic frequencies.
2. Lightworkers tune into the circulation of the collective higher consciousness.
3. Lightworkers are 100 percent committed to personal growth no matter what; it is kind of like an addiction (I am writing this at 3:23 a.m.; I know this info is needed right now).
4. Lightworkers believe in miracles.
5. Lightworkers work with energy flow and synchronicities.
6. Lightworkers sense the need to help and heal people.
7. Lightworkers have a close connection with the universe and energy.
8. Lightworkers are manifesters of power who know how to access their superpowers.

As the planet's consciousness rises, so does yours. You may start to feel some of these traits in your body. Your awareness is growing, and you are opening up to advances you have never heard of before, looking for opportunities to do something new and different. This time, you want to get it right—not follow in other people's footsteps but create a trailblazing path that is all yours. Not anyone else's.

Types of lightworkers and luminaries:

1. Celestial Luminaries: These luminaries maintain higher vibrational patterns and frequencies. Think of them as human lighthouses. Their job is to shine their light and give you hope, uplift and support you as you go through this awakening process of remembering who you really are. They bring higher vibration to the planet in the form of comedy, laughter, motivation, and spiritual teachers.

2. The Curers: The curers are healers who help with every single thing: all beings, all souls, Mother Nature, the animal kingdom, and mankind. These curers heal all beings mentally, emotionally, energetically, physically, and spiritually. By listening to their inner compass, they flow with the energy and align with frequencies to gain information on new healing modalities, techniques, and ways of using these gifts of service. They raise their vibration to heal, serve, love, support, and guide others to more fulfilling lives.

3. The Fantasizers: Fantasizers go into surreal dream space, which allows them to levitate into dimensions of experience, feelings, and visions. They connect to unique ideas to encourage and motivate the human soul. Almost all of the technology, art, and inventions we have in the world today come from the fantasizers.

4. The Gateways: These workers generate the human grid that links the hearts of all beings that have been awakened. The gateways are portals that link ley lines and act as doorways to allow light to come to this world through their open hearts.

5. Blueprint Keepers: Blueprint keepers are the receivers of the sacred codes for awakening. By translating the universal language codes, such as sacred geometry, they allow everyone to understand them and use them to raise levels of consciousness. Each person has their own blueprint, and when fully activated and awakened, they become the highest version of themselves, raising conscious awakening for humanity.

6. The Forecasters: These lightworkers have activated their third eye, which I call the invisible information station. Their expanded insight allows them to see beyond the physical and illusions. They are here to guide you to your truth by helping to inspire and empower you to listen to your inner intuition. Forecasters disclose the truth behind the shadows.

7. The Ambassadors: Ambassadors receive guidance from their higher self, cosmos, source, and higher realms. You may have encountered them through YouTube, podcasts, social media platforms, and literature. Ambassadors serve mankind in transition—in the process of obtaining enlightenment—by sharing powerful wisdom, be it through blogging, teaching, writing, videos, webinars, or seminars. They explain what is happening from their perspective so we can better understand the evolution of this planet and our soul purpose.

8. Timeline Transformers: These workers convert darkness and negative energy into light by releasing their energy to help restore balance. Timeline transformers work on behalf of the collective consciousness of humanity, transforming karma of the past. Some may also transform ancestral lines; born into ancestral lines riddled with negative karma, they serve, release, and heal their line in order to level up their vibration, also known as timeline healing. Timeline healing is one of the most super-powerful things you can do for the entire universe.

9. Light Manifesters: These lightworkers manifest profound changes by interlacing light into the community as a whole. They thereby shed light on darkness and can alter timelines and generate productive events and optimistic energies for creation of extraordinary love and vibrant harmony. Light manifesters generate the highest vibration of humanity and the universe.

10. Ascension Conductors: They teach the ascension process by moving into the light. We are all here to ascend. Ascension

conductors propel us to the next awakened level. They will help push the spiritual evolution of humanity. They approach from a higher perspective, looking for hazards that might not appear on the surface.

11. The Pavers: Pavers can see into someone else's heart and remind them of what they are here to do. The pavers personify the ascension process and live their lives in a unique authentic way. By living an enlightened and inspired life, they prioritize the interests of all beings, knowing full well they are here to serve humanity. The pavers pave the path of living in resonance with their truth and share their teachings with the world, teaching us nonattachment and reminding us of what really matters to the soul.

12. The Connectors: The connectors see and feel how everything links together. They notice patterns, mix philosophies, and can translate teachings of other lightworkers and shape the information so it is easy for people to consume. Connectors combine lightworkers of different types so their influence comprises a greater force on the planet.

How to tell if you are a lightworker or luminary:

1. You are always seeking deeper self-awareness and awareness of life in general.
2. You are an extremely powerful creator and manifester.
3. What you focus on creates results (so make sure your power is headed in the right direction).
4. You resonate energy, ascension, and ancient spirituality.
5. You can be psychic when it comes to what other people need, think, or are feeling in order to heal.

6. You know you are here to do the work and terminate old karmic patterns, cracking open a new level of awareness and consciousness.

7. Self-growth is your passion.

8. You feel strong ties with Mother Nature, intuitively knowing she aligns us to source the fastest.

9. You have experienced an intense or multiple awakenings that have propelled you to shatter your world and rebuild it again, which can be a painful and exhausting process.

10. You sense you are part of a global effort to raise the world's consciousness and are a "trailblazer" or "frontrunner" in the community.

11. You intuitively know you are alive to serve a higher purpose—one that involves transforming your life and the lives of others by helping raise the collective consciousness of humanity.

12. You have possessed wisdom since you were young and are highly intuitive.

13. You are a bit of a loner. Being in your own energy is healthier, since you are sensitive to other people's energy and can only take it in small amounts.

14. Your life was set up for heartache, trauma, difficulty, and challenges that were intended not to hurt you but to arouse the healer in you.

15. When it comes to mental illness, you now understand that you were adapting to your situation rather than being the problem itself. Helping revolutionize the way people witness emotional, mental, physical, and spiritual health transcends humanity.

## I Am a Luminary

I believe I am a luminary lightworker and was for many years before I even realized it. In 2014 I created a film called *Luminary*, dedicated to reincarnation, and it is about the light within.

The epiphanies hitting me back-to-back as I write this book have been extraordinary and surreal. There were days I cried at the vastness of information and energies pouring out of me and onto these pages. The ideas flowed faster than I could comprehend them until they moved through my body and the visualizations took place. This information can alter mankind for the better if you are ready to receive it. And I truly believe you are ready now. I feel so blessed to have had all these experiences and accomplishments to share with you.

This is my gift to the world: to teach you and show you how we all can communicate as one. When I read the luminary/lightworker types and descriptions, I realize I am a combination of all of them to a certain extent. That is how I was able to generate this book. I can condense a lot of complex information and bring it down to a level of greater understanding.

Many other people have these capabilities and have been greatly overlooked. These people are now coming to the surface and stepping up to share their knowledge with you. We are here to guide you and help you open up to other realms, densities, energies, and frequencies. You will do this by clearing the toxins out of your body, healing your inner self, realigning your biofield, and using senses you didn't know existed. You are a superpower. Get ready to clear stuck energy in the body and heal parts of your soul. The mission here is to heal so you can be one with everyone as we create one of the greatest highest vibrational frequencies of superpower life forces on this planet. Heaven on earth.

• • •

# HEALERS AND EXPERTS TO LEARN FROM

The following are healers I have learned from, worked with, listened to, researched, and watched for many years. The journey of a lightworker/luminary is the road less traveled and is often met with resistance. In the beginning, they were often shunned or even sued for healing people no other doctor could. Now the new-earth order is opening up and a super shift is taking place to open the gateway to bring these healing modalities into our pipeline. These incredible resources will magnify our ability to amp our superpowers to amazing heights. Humanity is evolving on a whole new level. This is where science and spirit connect. We will heal the body, heart, mind, and soul with sound, science, energy, frequency, and technology.

Many of the healers below offer training, creating new opportunities for new-earth professions. I offer this knowledge to the younger generations who have come here to heal mankind and alter our course in the universe.

## Bill McKenna: Cognomovement

https://www.Cognomovement.com

Cognomovement is a newer healing modality. I don't watch the news, but I am always watching shows and taking notes, and this was how I discovered cognomovement, created by Bill McKenna and Liz Larson. The premise involves using a volleyball with the colors and symbols of the chakras on the surface. Rotating it around your face, you use eye movement to tap into the subconscious and unconscious mind to gather information, new perspectives, and insights not found in everyday life.

People in the show stated they'd had a shift after one session. I found this concept rather interesting. I came across this particular show for a second time and felt the urge to watch again, which I don't normally do. I decided to see where Bill McKenna resided. It turned out he lived one county over from me. I reached out and spoke with a woman who said he was not available until the following week because he was prepping to lead a retreat at Mount Shasta. I have always wanted to go to Mount Shasta—wish I'd caught onto the idea a little earlier.

I was eager to talk to a practitioner just to pick their brain. I pulled up the cognomovement website and found a list. Knowing full well many of them were probably going to the retreat, I decided to call a few, getting the feeling that the right one would answer the phone and have the information that I needed to hear. And that is exactly what happened. A woman by the name of Annette picked up the phone, and we conversed for about an hour. Her knowledge, experience, and guidance was edifying, and we had a great connection. She filled me in on the benefits her clients received from their cognomovement sessions. She talked about the biofield meter and being able to read people's energy around the body. Annette encouraged me to partake in cognomovement, claiming people she knew had completely changed their lives for the better from their sessions.

I ended up booking an appointment to meet with Bill McKenna the following week since he was just about an hour's drive away. Bill directed me to come right to his house, and we worked for several hours on deep-rooted issues in my family timeline.

You see, things from our childhood that we don't get clarity on can stick with us for eternity if we don't do something about it. My father had died when I was a young girl from alcoholism. I truly believe he died from a broken heart. He was a misunderstood, spiritual man and had turned to drinking to numb his senses, as a lot of sensitive people do. When alcohol took over his life, I suffered in many ways from his unpredictability. But when he died, I knew he had become my guardian angel.

In time, I had a very hard time trusting men in general. I had no problem getting a date or finding men who wanted to spend time with me, but their main motivation was sex and siphoning my life force. They didn't want to know, love, or accept the real me. So I started to steer clear of men. When I had my session with Bill, I had a breakthrough moment in the midst of tears and deep healing. You see, when you use cognomovement, your eyes move back and forth, bringing messages into your body and brain, connecting the subconscious and unconscious mind, about what you need to do for you. I would say it's like getting a phone call from your higher self.

I discovered my dad drank himself to death because he couldn't stand not being with his kids and family. My stepfather had moved in and taken over the house my dad built and his blood family; it was the ultimate pain for my dad to watch and bear. He just couldn't get over it, and it drew him into a spiral of pain and depression, which led him to drink more and lose his bearings. In that session, I got the sense that my dad had decided to let himself die. Because he couldn't be with us in real life, he died so he could always watch over us from the other side. It was his ultimate sacrifice in order to stay connected to us no matter what. I always knew in my heart he was there for me. But hearing and feeling it from him made it that much clearer and more impactful.

Cognomovement can be used to break a habit, change the way you feel about your body, or heal deep emotions. All you have to do is focus on the issue and use the step-by-step movements to get to the root. I do believe that in the future we will see cognomovement centers, and therapists will incorporate cognomovement into their sessions if they are smart and really looking toward the true light of helping people heal on all levels.

I purchased the cognomovement ball and attended a few learning sessions. That ball comes in very handy when I am feeling unsettled with anything in my life. In one instance, when I was really struggling with my health, I picked up that ball for a few minutes; that is when I got the message that I needed to heal from the inside out and that I needed to get good water, which started me on my journey to finding the best water on the planet, which led me to PEMF therapy, which lead me to better nutrition.

Cognomovement moves energy within the body, accelerating healing on multiple levels. As simple as it seems, using a combination of healing modalities to peel back the layers of trauma and internal scarring releases and helps you open up to other perspectives that allow you to forgive and heal. Cognomovement has been used to help children heal as well. It's an easy method to bring into schools, communities, and senior centers. You will most likely feel a shift right away; during the days that follow, more radical shifts may occur, bringing new light to a situation.

In another cognomovement session, I got the urge to write and complete this book. I acted on it immediately but was quickly overtaken by my job, which didn't leave me the energy to allow the book to surface properly. I told Annette about my internal knowing that I was supposed to finally write a book. As of today, I still have not met Annette in person since she lives in another state. She doesn't even know I'm in the process of writing this book. In fact, as of this very moment of writing, I have told no one about this book. I have just allowed it to manifest freely and without anyone else's input. I have done this on purpose so that only my energy emits from this book. I am sure Annette will be ecstatic when she hears what has transpired from yet another cognomovement session.

Cognomovement is holistic healing on the cutting edge. Therapist, coaches, and counselors: we need you to add this to your services. It's an entirely new take on clearing energy and understanding the world at large.

Keeping a journal of your sessions is beneficial. This way you can go back and refer to the sensations and feelings you received when you worked through your issue.

You never know what new healing technique will be on the horizon. Technology and humans are evolving at an extremely accelerated rate, bringing in a new frontier of opportunities to heal yourself. Stay open to these new-earth ideas, and you might just find the exact thing to propel you into an advanced state of mind you never thought you could reach.

Cognomovement is accelerated learning, which means accelerated healing.

## Dylan Varenhorst, the Spirit Advisor: Human Design Master, Cognition Coach

https://www.HDmaven.com

Dylan is one of my best kept secrets. I met Dylan at a yoga event and was mesmerized by his vast knowledge. Dylan is not your typical human in his thirties. He operates on a level I have never seen before from anyone and is a true leader of civilization for the younger generations to follow. Living a life of simplicity and observation, connecting with energetic frequencies, working in the quantum fields, and connecting dots from other dimensions, he will propel you to a level of understanding and perception you never knew existed.

Dylan will glean insights about you by reading the quantum blueprint of your soul. He truly is "the spirit advisor." Utilizing your birthday, birth time, and birth location to generate your Human Design blueprint, he will be able to tell you unusual things about your DNA and genetic makeup that reveal what you are meant to do on this planet. He will basically give you your life map. Turn your limited time on this planet into unlimited possibilities by learning and owning who you are.

Dylan helped me see, feel, and generate this book years ago by insights he gave me along the way. I just had to get out of my own way, remove the obstacles, and do the work. Dylan is here to help children and their families discover who they are and teach them how to become the best versions of themselves.

## Larisa Stow: Lead Singer of Shakti Tribe, Sound Healer, Coach

https://www.LarisaStow.com

I met Larisa at the yoga retreat in Joshua Tree National Forest when I was just beginning my deep healing journey. I think the universe really wanted me there. Larisa helped me heal chakras in my body through the vibration of sound, movement, music, mantras, and energy. I will never forget my first encounter and experience with her.

She had us dive deep within our soul to tap into stuck energy in the body. We each partnered up with a person we didn't know. Holding our hands together, we sat cross-legged, singing face-to-face. When I looked at the girl across from me, she didn't turn away. She looked directly into my soul. It was the first time I felt like anybody really saw my soul and accepted me for who I was. Tears streamed down my face when I realized this stranger loved me unconditionally. My body, heart, and soul released and accepted this woman's energy. She filled me up with acceptance, health, well-being, compassion, and love. Tears come to my eyes as I write this when I recall the feelings she bestowed upon me—a true gift of an incredible energy exchange.

After the event, I walked up to Larisa and told her about my experience. She asked me where I lived because she felt compelled to help me. Turns out she didn't live far from me. I attended more events with Larisa. She taught us about the benefits of healing waters, grounding, releasing energy, exchanging energy, vibrational healing, Reiki healing, and other energetic body components. Larisa has traveled all over the world and worked with all kinds of resources and healers, becoming a healing source of her own power.

While I was going through my divorce, I came in a complete shaking mess. Larisa directed the entire group to surround me and lay their hands on me. I cried uncontrollably as they poured their loving energy into me while taking the negative energy out.

I introduce you to vibrational sound healer Larisa Stow. She most definitely belongs in this lineup. My goal is to bring her in on events so you all can get to know her and feel her radiant love and vibrational frequencies and partake in her magic. Larisa leads retreats around the world and offers a unique modality.

## Christian Reid: Sound Healer

https://www.Soundbathsandyoga.com

The power of sound is part of our new-earth push toward conscious expansion and healing fragments of the soul, and I believe it to be humanity's ultimate healing tool.

Christian's sound bath was the first I ever attended. Right then and there, I realized the power of sound. I felt it in my head, heart, chakras, meridians, teeth, bones, blood, and body on a cellular level. And I want you to understand that not all sound baths are alike. Each person is going to bring something different to the table, depending on their energy, their awareness, and their ability to expand and help you expand. A sound bath practitioner has to be able to completely let go and surrender to higher frequencies and bring them toward you. I have been to many sound baths and have had excellent results. However, Christian's methods worked the best for me on a higher level—by far.

This man uses a large variety of instruments, including his voice. His is the voice of the past, present, and future when combined with his techniques. Changing of the vocal chords with air alters both the level and frequency spectrum of voice sound. This opens up the gateway to speech intelligibility, which can flood a person with the highest wisdom, knowledge, visions, insights, and all knowing.

The sound and character of the voice is unique to each person. I am all about listening to someone's voice. A lot of information is projected: how they think, feel, and analyze life. When considering meeting someone from an online dating app, I've always made it a point to talk to them on the phone first. I want to gauge how their voice makes me feel. Does it calm me or annoy me? Can they hold a conversation? Are they interesting or sarcastic? Many people just want to text endlessly. Who has time for that? Texting is such a waste of life force energy and time if you ask me. I want to live in the moment, exchanging energy.

Some dating apps have added the option to record a voice message so people can listen. Voice recordings don't sound entirely the same as someone does live, but you can still get a reading off their voice.

Several times after attending Christian's sound bath events, I had monumental shifts. I didn't even tell Christian until years later when I ran into him again. He had no idea and was so surprised to hear the good news. I wanted him to know his healing affected me in a very positive way and to keep up the good work.

I am all about affirming people. When you do this, you lift your frequency as well as theirs to another level. After all, the name of the game on this planet is leveling up. Christian offers lessons to those looking to learn this skill set; just check out his website. You can follow Christian on Instagram and purchase his music as well. But if you ever get the opportunity to hear him live, I say dive in and get ready to be taken into the next dimension.

## David Elliot: Breathwork Teacher, Author, and Healer

https://www.davidelliott.com

It took me several years to discover the man who taught me how to be a breathwork guide. I knew I wanted to learn it, but life is all about timing of the universe.

David hosts weekend retreats that lead us into deeper levels of healing in multiple realms and dimensions. We spend the days uprooting what needs to be cleared by bringing it to the surface. It is very emotional and intense at times because we are digging up our own dirt. When conversing with David on one of these retreats, I could sense his sensitivity to my pent-up energy. I was just hitting the tip of the iceberg, and he knew it.

The weekend workshops run several weekends, months apart. We expand in between sessions and come back together to release, learn, and evolve.

David has helped many famous people in the Los Angeles area and carries a very calming frequency. He is a great teacher and leader in the realm of holistic health. Many people return over and over to his events to continue to grow, stay connected, and hone their skills. If you are looking to learn the technique of breathwork or become a practitioner, David Elliot is your guy. Breathwork is utilized in drug and alcohol recovery centers as a way to heal and move energy.

## Sandhiya Ramaswamy: Ayurveda Nutritional Coach

https://www.alchemyayurveda.com

Sandhiya is a monumental life force. She transformed my mind, body, and soul with the proper nutrition my body needed to achieve amazing health. Sandhiya gave me the eleven-page questionnaire I talked about earlier that asked me more health questions than a doctor's form. She offers one-on-one consultations, cooking classes, online courses, and retreats.

I found Sandhiya at a yoga center I didn't even attend. I walked in and found Ayurveda products on the shelf and asked if they knew of an Ayurveda nutritionist. Talk about timing of the universe. I was on the lookout for a good one, and then she surfaced. Little did I know she was above and beyond what I expected. I share this great resource with you in hopes of helping you transform your life with this results-oriented life-health coach.

## Billy Carson: Financial Strategist, Author

https://www.4biddenknowledge.com

I discovered Mr. Carson on TV, where he talked about the financial matrix. His ideas and theories fascinated me, and I felt very much in alignment with many of his teachings. He talked of legacy building, manifesting, passion, setting up future generations, an abundance mindset, and envisioning, to name a few topics. I also caught him on other shows, talking about UFOs and ancient civilizations. Being a huge fan of history, I was hooked. Mr. Carson provides fresh perspectives backed by evidence and is definitely someone you will want to check out.

## Caroline Cory: Superhuman: *The Invisible Made Visible*

https://www.CarolineCory.com

I love this lady. She is sharing it all with you and me, providing scientific evidence to get the nonbelievers to see and comprehend. I love *Superhuman* and recommend you go check it out if you are looking to make a radical shift in perspective.

## Eileen McKusick: Creator of Biofield Tuning, Author

https://www.biofieldtuning.com, https://www.electrichealth.com

Eileen is a researcher, writer, inventor, practitioner, educator, and speaker on the effect of audible sound on the human body and biofield. She is the inventor of the sonic slider tool and CEO of BioSana, which provides sound therapy tools.

A few days after I got the message to add the section on sound healing to this book, I listened to the Science of Healing Summit on the Shift Network and came across Eileen. The universe literally lined up the right minds to help me connect the dots to share them with you.

Eileen is in the fields of therapeutic sound and electric health. She is founder of the Biofield Tuning Institute, so if this type of work resonates with you, you can become a practitioner and learn more by visiting her website.

## Jeralyn Glass: Sound Healer

https://www.jeralynglass.com

Jeralyn is taking sound healing into another dimension by communicating through sound with her deceased son. She uses advanced singing bowls infused with crystal energies, enabling her to reach higher frequencies of communication. She is an internationally known singer, professor, meditation leader, sound-healing practitioner, and crystal singing bowl master alchemist. Jeralyn blends her love for music and frequency, teaching other practitioners to do the same.

## John Stuart Reid: Acoustics Scientist, Inventor of the CymaScope

https://www.cymascope.com, https://www.soundmadevisible.com

Thank you, John, for the invention of the CymaScope. Cymatics is the science of visible vibrations and sound, and John is leading the way to educate and inspire the world on his findings. His CymaScope invention has forever changed the world's perception of sound by giving us the ability to "see" sound and vibration and better understand this super shift. Sound is revealed in a myriad of geometric patterns. As I have such a strong connection to sacred geometry and mathematics, it makes complete sense to me.

If you want to learn cutting-edge information on the frequency of sound, follow this guy. He is going where no man has gone before.

## Nick Ortner: Author of *The Tapping Solution*

https://www.thetappingsolution.com

In 2013, Nick Ortner wrote a book educating others on "the tapping solution." In 2021 and 2022, he offered the Tapping World Summit, which is a free online training event introducing others to tapping. I participated. He had guest speakers, authors, and influencers sharing their strategies and techniques for all to learn from at no cost.

You can also purchase the Tapping Solution app to pull up anytime, should the need to do a tapping session on yourself or someone else arise. This is some pretty powerful information we all can have and do on our own for very little cost. Thank you, Nick Ortner.

## Wendie Colter: Medical Intuitive Training, Founder/CEO of the Practical Path, Inc.

https://www.thepracticalpath.com

Wendie Colter is founder and CEO of the Practical Path, Inc. She offers intuitive development programs for wellness professionals and the general public. Wendie has her own accredited certification program for medical intuitive training, which has been monumental in helping holistic health professionals from every walk of life expand their intuition.

Wendie teaches how to read other people's energy with your eyes closed, purely by tapping into the energy field and source. She has been asked to bring her teachings to traditional medicine practices so traditional doctors can incorporate them. I believe Wendie's medical intuitive training will be part of the trend toward combining holistic health perspectives with traditional medicine.

## Bradley Nelson: The Emotion Code

https://www.HealersLibrary.com, https://www.DiscoverHealing.com

The Body Code is a revolutionary energy-balancing system intended to help you uncover root causes of discomfort, sickness, and suffering in body and spirit. It is an extensive natural energy-healing tool that can be utilized through an app on your phone. By answering a series of questions while doing muscle testing, one can often identify what is happening in the body that needs attention.

Our amazing bodies move through the world by releasing and contracting muscles. The body's cells know their entire history and what the body needs to acquire in order to regain full health. Muscle testing retrieves knowledge imbedded in the cellular memory of the muscular system and pinpoints energy blockages. During the test, gentle pressure is applied to points in the muscular system while the participant is asked questions, generating biofeedback on the body's physiological and psychological state. By the process of elimination, we can home in on the one component the body needs to regain full health alignment.

DNA is influenced by different signals from outside the cell. Our thoughts, attitudes and beliefs are the strongest energetic signals that cells receive. By controlling our mindfulness, we can control how our bodies respond. It can be a simple as adding a supplement that the body is low on, or the body might require more complex rebalancing. Emotion code helps with emotional wellness, body system balance, toxin resolution, pathogen resolution, structural balance, nutrition, and lifestyle. Are you noticing a pattern here? We keep coming back to nutrition and lifestyle.

Many people suffer from emotional baggage that is stuck in the body and needs to be cleared to create the life we want. If we don't clear it, this causes illness in the body. By understanding and moving the energy of emotions through the body, you can realign your system. All you have to do is ask for help, and the subconscious mind will open you up to what is going on.

By connecting the physical body with the spirit, we can also help release baggage we are dragging around from our ancestors. When we release inherited trapped emotions, there is a ripple effect, called timeline healing—transformational experience for the living as well as for those who have passed.

## Dr. Joe Dispenza

https://www.Drjoedispenza.com

Dr. Dispenza is a researcher, consultant, author, and educator who has traveled to over thirty-three countries, lecturing on how to discover the full potential of the human brain and how to use it for personal development. I have seen him on TV shows, heard him on YouTube, and follow him on Instagram. I have pages and pages of written notes from his segments. His insights are extraordinary. He has taught over 50,000 people and has three *New York Times* bestsellers to his name. Search him online to connect to his meditations, books, and resources.

## Bruce H. Lipton, PhD: Epigenetics, Cellular Biologist, Author

https://www.BruceLipton.com

Epigenetics is the study of cellular and physiological traits—specifically, how environmental factors and behavior affect our genes and define how our cells behave. Bruce's premise is that the emotions in the body dictate how the body and brain chemistry respond and create on a cellular level.

Bruce Lipton calls out the pharmaceutical industry. The concept behind epigenetics is that you can alter your genetics by modifying your behavior rather than taking medications. By incorporating the concepts I have shared in this book, such as switching to living water, consuming nutritional products, getting proper sleep, detoxing the body, controlling your mindset, and reprogramming the mind, you can become your super self.

I have caught Bruce a couple of times on several different TV shows. This man is well known in the field of epigenetics and has podcasts, webinars, books, and a monthly newsletter you can subscribe to learn more detailed information.

## Gregg Braden: The Wisdom Codes

https://www.greggbraden.com

Gregg Braden is a five-time *New York Times* bestselling author, scientist, and educator. Gregg merges science, social policy, and human potential in his research.

Gregg breaks the codes on biology and neurosciences, revealing how the structure of language—the words we think and speak—can actually change the way the neurons in our brains and heart connect. So be very careful what you say. Our ancestors intuitively understood these connections thousands of years ago and created specific word patterns to provide healing, comfort, and inner power in difficult times. By encoding powerful words in prayers, we can become better, healed versions of ourselves.

## Dr. Alberto Villoldo: Author of *Grow a New Body: How Spirit and Power Plant Nutrients Can Transform Your Health*

https://www.thefourwinds.com, https://www.albertovilloldophd.com, https://www.growanewbody.com

Alberto Villoldo, PhD, is a medical anthropologist and has studied shamanic healing practices of the Amazon and Andes for more than thirty years. As founder of the Four Winds Society, he combines modern medicine with ancient shamanic traditions.

It all comes down to detoxification, and Dr. Alberto Villoldo has the resources to back it up. When you heal, you retain youthful vitality, which helps you keep connected to the earth and your purpose in life. Food is part of the fountain of youth. Nutrition is one of the fastest ways to gain your health back. Food is medicine.

The new world will consist of preparing traditional medicine practitioners with shamanic education in order to disseminate wise and ethical energy medicine practices on this planet.

## Donna Eden: Author of *Energy Medicine*

https://www.edenmethod.com, https://www.learnenergymedicine.com

Donna Eden is a spokesperson for energy medicine and one of the most vibrant people of her time. She can "see" the body's energies, and her abilities as a healer are one of a kind. Her bestselling book *Energy Medicine* is the textbook in hundreds of healing classes and is available in twenty languages. Donna and her husband, David Feinstein, have built the world's largest organization that teaches hands-on use of energy medicine. They have 1,600 certified practitioners and serve clients all over the US, Canada, Latin America, Europe, Asia, and Australia. These healers are trailblazers bringing in the new-earth order.

## Lynne McTaggart: Author of *What Doctors Don't Tell You, The Intention Experiment, The Field, The Bond,* and *The Power of Eight*

https://www.lynnemctaggart.com

Lynne McTaggart, an authority on the new science of consciousness, has now had her books translated into thirty languages. She orchestrates intention experiments, which are web-based "global laboratory" experiments, to test the power of intention to heal the world. A highly sought-after public speaker, Lynne has been listed by Peter Russell as one of the 100 most spiritually influential living people. How is that for impact?

## Rollin McCraty, PhD: Director of Research at HeartMath Institute

https://www.heartmath.org

Rollin McCraty, PhD, is a psychophysiologist whose interests include the physiology of emotion, focusing on how emotions influence mental processing, behavior, and health and the global interconnectivity between people and the earth's energetic systems. Rollin has investigated the effects of emotions on heart–brain interactions and on cardiovascular, hormonal, immune system, and autonomic function.

• • •

# IN CONCLUSION

Every day, new discoveries are being made, and the field of holistic health is ever evolving. It is exciting, cutting-edge, and advanced technology for humankind. I invite you to continue diving into these realms to discover them for yourself.

The ultimate goal is to create the highest vibrational frequency we can on this planet, on our way to reach ascension.

> **JOURNAL: Chapter 10**
>
> 1. Write in your journal any of these soul-healing techniques that interest you.
> 2. Research the techniques by visiting the links or researching them on your own so you can expand your awareness. Add any good notes you learn along the way into your journal. You are building your own book of knowledge on topics that comprise the new world as we know it.

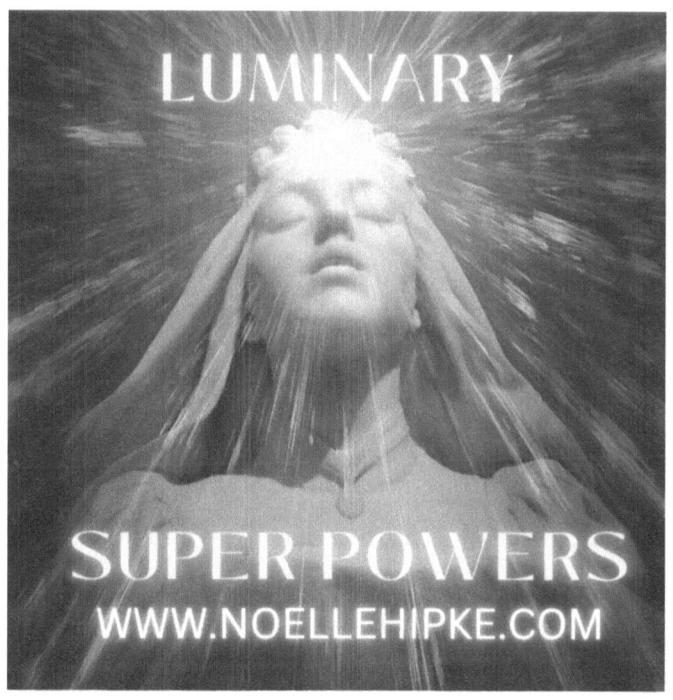

## CHAPTER 11

# WRAP-UP

Here is all the information I hope you internalize:

- **Extrasensory Perception (ESP)**: Tap into extraordinary senses you didn't even know existed by detoxing.

- **Dial Perception**: Use your ears and head glands to pick up invisible information. Your body and head can sense things miles away like an animal does. Again, you need to be toxin-free. This term dial perception came to me in a dream, asking me to share this expanded perception with you.

- **Sleep**: Sleep helps heal the cells and regenerates skin, organs, eyes, bones, etc. Sleep is the fountain of youth. Dreaming enables you to travel into other dimensions where you gather information. It comes in the form of colors, numbers, feelings, symbols, people, and objects. You can astral travel, transcend, and get messages from your higher self. Keep a physical, written dream journal and look up meanings to interpret.

- **Higher Self**: Your higher self is a part of your soul living in a higher dimension. It gathers multiple aspects from other realms you cannot see or hear. Your higher soul self sends messages to you through meditation, quiet time, and relaxation, in the shower, while journaling or connecting to nature, during exercise, and through feelings, dreams, symbols, synchronies, and the mind, body, and gut. Tapping into your body gives you the info you need. Quiet your mind and listen. Ask yourself a question, and your higher self will answer.

- **World Travel**: Watch and study cultures around the world. Many other cultures travel widely, speak multiple languages, and have long-standing traditions that should be respected and honored. Their ancestors created these traditions for good reasons. We should not judge people because they are different or have different coloring or beliefs. Traditions carry potent knowledge and medicine. We should always consider new options and learn from one another. We are all equal as one. When we unite, we are one of the most powerful electrical forces in the universe.

- **Torus Field**: Time travel/space travel/torus travel can be achieved when working in the higher consciousness realms of the fourth dimensions and above. Tied into sacred geometry, the energies of the human body can be aligned to higher states of being to access unlimited knowledge from universal energy flow, granting messages from the chalice of the Holy Grail and connecting you directly to the divine source, God.

- **Astral Travel**: Astral travel is also known as astral projection, which enables you to move the soul out of your body to travel around the universe energetically without the need for a body. This type of travel gives you unlimited information as you move through the holographic and quantum fields.

- **Remote Viewing**: Remote viewing enables you to move between different points using mental imagery; for example, you can take a look around a geographic landmark, event, object or person on the other side of the earth.

- **Auras**: Auras are seen as bubbles that reflect the vibrational energy of every living being—including plants, animals, and even Mother Nature herself—and come in different strengths and colors.

- **Biofield**: The biofield is the energy field that surrounds and extends out from the body around eight feet and can be felt with the hands through pressure and temperature changes. The biofield is composed of measurable electromagnetic energy, chi, and subtle energy.
- **Clairsentience**: Clear feeling.
- **Claircognizance**: Clear knowing.
- **Clairvoyance**: Clear seeing.
- **Clairalience**: Clear smelling.
- **Clairaudience**: Clear hearing.
- **Clairgustance**: Clear tasting.
- **Telepathy**: Flash perception.
- **Transcendence**: Rising above.
- **New Earth**: We can create change for the better for you, your children, and humankind. You are the future of Planet Earth. You have the power to create greatness and beauty in the world. Use your superpowers to heal, help, and raise each other's vibrations. Act in positive ways for the planet and each other. Create a world where we combine resources, thoughts, and beliefs and cultivate oneness.
- **Ancestral DNA**: Change the children, and we change the lineage of past, present, and future generations. We do this by identifying behaviors and changing the way we think, perceive, accept, decide, behave, and judge. What has been imbedded in our DNA affects our unconscious and subconscious minds. This is how parents pass down lineage problems and negative behaviors. Healing our DNA is crucial to breaking the cycle. Use healing methods in this book to clear and heal yourself, and watch and feel the magic take place.

- **Journal**: Journal to release and see a pattern. Read, learn, watch, listen, and witness. Journaling frees the mind and gives it space to let patterns go and recreate new ones. Emotions are released; stuck energy is released. Have a journal for gratitude, a journal for releasing, and a journal for creating. Start a journaling club. Sit in silence out in nature while you each write. Come back in a group circle and share any insights you want to manifest as a group, be it world peace, health, or success; working in after-school groups amplifies superpowers.

- **Nutrition**: Food is medicine, food is energy, and food is information. When you eat fresh, organic foods from healthy soil or without pesticides or antibiotics, your body takes on superpower energy from the food. Light codes of information and healing come from the sun, so when you put fresh, healthy fruits and veggies into your body, this activates your superpowers, force field, and biofield and allows a super shift. Grow your own garden if you have a yard, and put the most precious food you can create in your own body. When you eat like this, you vibrate higher and can reach higher levels of knowledge, wisdom, and an all-knowing universal energy flow.

- **Nutritional Reset**: When I was going through a monumental healing period, I came across one of the purest nutritional products I had ever found. I tried this product for several months before I decided to present it to the outside world. I had some major detoxing to do since I had never done a detox in my life. I sought products that would help me go holistic and natural and carried the highest vibration ingredients found on the planet. Nutrition helps people get their health back in record time.

  Nutritional reset gets metals and toxins out of the body, which assists with memory, the thyroid, menopause, diabetes, cancer, organs, brain fog, and other health issues people suffer from. Using natural nutrition enhances the human body, working on the cellular level to get your body into peak states. I was able to get off prescription drugs for my thyroid by replacing them with natural nutritional supplements. And when I learned nutritional reset helps women in menopause and assists people with weight loss and belly fat, I knew it was a force for good.

We all need to fill in the gap with vitamins and supplements. There is no possible way to eat healthy all the time. And if we don't have access to the foods our body needs, using these supplements are a great way to tap into our superpowers. I am more than happy to offer you guidance on the best products to suit your unique situation, and I recommend you also work with a nutritionist to create the best scenario for your body, mind, and soul. Our soul-healing journey really ties into what we put into our bodies and how we connect all the components to work together in harmony. You can gain access to more information and recommendations through my website at https://www.LuminaryHealingCenter.com and reach out for a custom consultation.

- **Detention**: Kids in detention are in detention because something is not right in their home or personal or school life. They are not being heard, respected, understood, or guided. These kids need a mentor to help them identify the root cause and discover what will help them thrive, feel alive, and light up.

- **Grounding**: Every day, go out in nature and walk barefoot or lie on the ground, grass, sand, or dirt. This will help align your body to Mother Nature's rhythms, remove stuck energy, bring in good energy, and open you up to universal energy flow. Universal energy flow contains knowledge and healing. This helps prevent illness, keeps you connected, and removes radiation from 5G and other devices we are surrounded by on a daily basis.

- **Social Media/News Media**: Control the data coming into your brain, body, and environment. It affects you invisibly—energetically, emotionally, physically, and mentally. Do not share personal information online that you don't want the entire world and universe to know. Once is it out there, it is tattooed on you. Do not partake in bashing, bullying, or rejection on social media. This could create karma you don't want.

- **Digital Matrix**: Get out of the digital matrix at all costs when you can. Limit access to energies hijacking your brain, body, and biofield. Jobs, careers, and school will require you to work in the digital matrix in your lifetime. I have found that certain parts of the digital matrix deplete me of my life force energy. This happens when you play video games, go on Instagram, TikTok, etc. You are using your life force to engage with that game/platform. You are powering the program. You know the saying "The eyes are the windows to the soul"? Well, it holds true. These devices are reading and extracting your life force through your eyes and mind—hence telepathic suggestions from your devices on a subject you were thinking about.

    I have witnessed many people change from interacting too often with the digital matrix; it leads to psychological and emotional issues, suicide, and a slew of other negative situations. Going outside and being in nature will help you balance out these energies when you are subjected to them for the long term. You have got to release and get away from the radiation, mind control, and toxic messages being forced upon you. I was alive before the internet existed, and we didn't have mental and emotional issues like we do today. Sure, you can say I am old fashioned and don't know anything, like all teens want to believe about their parents. But I do know that the digital matrix is invisible poison to our bodies and brains, even if you don't want to believe it.

I have the knowledge and wisdom to be able to step back and see it for what it really is: mind control over society. If we can learn to not depend on devices or be sold on the latest technology being cleverly marketed to us, we take back our power and gain control of our superpowers. Ignore this warning and you will be hijacked for your life force energy. Ultimately, the choice of what you will allow others to do to you is up to you.

- **Marijuana**: Marijuana is now legal. Why? Because it makes it easier to hijack your body and brain without you realizing it. When you are high, you are not living in the present moment, which makes it easier to steal your life force. I spent many years high and not feeling a thing. Boy, did I miss out on a lot of wonderful moments. Your subconscious and unconscious mind take over and lead the way, often not taking you in the direction you want to go. Intention is directional energy. And if you don't have any intention, you don't have any direction.

- **Electronic Devices**: Start to learn to live without devices—except to make phone calls, search the internet for projects only, and Zoom to connect with healthcare practitioners worldwide. You have the power of the worldwide web at your hands! Choose to use it wisely, and you will free yourself to discover what it truly means to live. These devices are sucking the superpowers, life force, and super shifts right out of you. If you want to research or look something up, write it in your journal and designate some future time to do the research. Completely turn off your devices at night and wipe them off with gloves and a cleaning cloth. Do not sleep with them at all; use a regular alarm clock. Being around these devices all the time is toxic for your mind and your body.

- **Superpowers**: You access and turn on your superpowers when you are aligned with yourself, eat a healthy diet, sleep, exercise, filter media, journal, meditate, and listen to your higher self. You are a force to be reckoned with when you are tapped in. Your superpowers are unique. There are things you will excel at over other people and vice versa. Honor, respect, and admire each other's unique superpowers. Stack your team with people of all different kinds of superpowers, and you will have the entire super package.

- **Super Shift**: A super shift occurs when you have accessed your superpowers and have maintained them at a high vibrational level for a decent period of time. You then move on to a higher frequency, which enables you to access new knowledge, understanding, and senses you never knew existed.

- **Force Field**: Your force field is the energetic biofield around your body. It represents the alignment of your chakras, meridians, and energy. Your force field can pick up invisible messages through observation, energy, vibrations, body language, emotions, feelings, senses, wavelengths, and your third eye (invisible information station).

- **Illness/Disability**: Illness is unhealed energy stuck in the body. If you have unresolved issues, are in a toxic situation or abusive relationship, or are replaying negative programming in the brain, this can cause sickness. We become what we believe, and if someone mistreats us or says hurtful things, we tend to play the scenario back in our heads like a recorded message. Reprogramming your brain, body, mind, feelings, and emotions in a positive light will help you heal and release the damage that has been done. You can heal yourself if you take the time to dig in, do the work, process, and push through the storm.

- **Bullies**: Bullies are people who hurt other people to make themselves feel better. Get out of any situation where someone starts instigating and attacking. Make up an excuse and leave the negative energy behind. No one wants to be affiliated with someone who is hurtful. Do not join in online conversations ripping people down. That negative energy could come back to haunt you.

- **Habits**: Modify your behavior to create healthy habits, and you have created a good, healthy lifestyle. You will be a role model for others to follow and look up to. Good habits define how you look, feel, and act.

- **Failure**: Fail every day. That means you tried and learned what works and doesn't work. You are developing your superpowers when you fail, by gaining knowledge and wisdom. If there is something that is too frustrating to deal with, walk away and accept the consequences of not accomplishing the task. Some things are just not worth sacrificing your soul, well-being, and happiness.

- **Common Sense**: Common sense is granted to those who put themselves out there even when they don't want to. You build up experience, knowledge, and wisdom as you journey through life. Mistakes need to be made to know right from wrong and to discover what works and what doesn't. Traveling accelerates common sense by enabling you to learn from people in other countries and other situations.

- **Intellect**: Intellect is acquired through reading, writing, observation, listening, asking questions, studying, hard work, understanding, learning for life, seminars, webinars, podcasts, books, workbooks, self-help, accepting and understanding others' differences, and creating win-win situations. Being intellectual can often mean being misunderstood, uncomfortable, and ultrasensitive to people, energy, emotions, vibrations, frequency, and invisible information. You are vibrating higher because you are tapped into higher dimensions of wisdom and knowledge not everyone can access. It can be very uncomfortable at times, but accept yourself, love yourself, understand yourself, and give yourself permission to be uniquely you.

- **Skin, Body, and Hair**: Your skin, eyes, hair, and the shape of your face and body has been picked out and designed especially just for you. You are beautiful. You are not supposed to look like or be like anybody else. Admire those who have different qualities than you. Do not be jealous. Honor and respect each person's superpowers, and hone and own yours. Loving yourself will draw the right people toward you. Surround yourself with people who make you feel good. You do not need to tan or change your body. Being the completely naturally you is part of the new world. Your body is an incredible healing machine that outlasts even stainless steel kitchen appliances. Think about that. How amazing are we? We need to thank our bodies for all the hard work they do. They will continue to treat us well if we treat them well.

- **Gratitude/Appreciation**: Gratitude and appreciation is a superpower that can manifest what you want in the present and future. By being grateful for what you have, you attract more love, kindness, health, and wealth. Remember: gratitude attitude.

- **Jealousy**: I do believe some people have jealousy imbedded in their DNA. They just can't help it, but they can be made aware of it and notice when they feel it and then decide how to act on it. It must be very hard to live with this emotion constantly eating at you. Forgive people who are jealous and move on. The issue is with them and not you. Don't be envious of what other people look like, what they have, or how successful they are. Each of us has our own problems, and what you see on the outside doesn't necessarily reflect the inside.

- **Anger/Frustration**: Don't be quick to get angry with others or judge. You do not know what they are dealing with. They could be struggling with serious emotional issues. Having kindness, compassion, forgiveness, and unconditional love is part of activating your superpowers. Give people peace and space. Do not explode and unload. Silence is often a superpower.

- **Release:** Forms of release include yelling, hollering, exercising, dancing, breathing, screaming, throwing, punching (punching bag), grounding, walking, running. Doing things that release and move the energy through your body helps clear, clean, and heal. Pushing it out and letting it go aligns you with universal energy flow.

- **Mind Mapping:** You can reprogram the brain with good thoughts while you exercise, training it to think, believe, and behave in a new way. Positive patterns are created in the central nervous system, in the cells, and in the brain, creating a better mindset. You may have to reprogram your brain on a daily basis, or reprogram it again after a traumatic incident. Reprogramming your brain will become a way of life.

- **Affirmations:** Write down, post, and record affirmations you want to program into your brain, body, and nervous system. Post the writings and read them out loud. Record them on your phone and listen to them when you walk, fold laundry, or meditate. Post them by your toilet so you can read and say them several times a day.

- **Guided Imagery:** Use guided imagery to create your future and heal your soul by creating time and space to become and accomplish what you want. Placing yourself in a situation you want to create puts you into vibration of making that event happen.

- **Vision Boards:** Create vision boards at the beginning of every year and hang them beside your bed. This way you see your vision every night before you go to sleep and every morning when you wake up. Keep your old visions boards; it may take a few years to completely manifest your idea, but you will want to look back and see what worked out.

- **Picnics**: Picnics are the secret to connecting to the earth with healing foods. Sit on the ground barefoot to gain the best possible healing. Eating healthy foods while vibrating and connecting to the earth puts you into ultimate high vibration. Spend a few hours doing this, and you will have the best sleep of your life.

- **Vibration**: Vibrations are the signals and frequencies of feelings and emotions you are sending out and receiving. Think of them as radio waves. Vibration determines how you are being heard in the world. What kind of messages are you sending out and receiving?

- **Sound Healing**: Musical instruments can heal your body on a cellular level. Sound harmonizes your cells to dance together and work in unison toward enhanced health. When under a deep sound-healing meditation, your body will clear energy, heal organs, send messages to the brain, and align your body and soul. This practice should be repeated over and over; it heals what needs to be healed at that moment in time. We pick up all sorts of energy on a daily basis, and we need to be able to clear it continuously. You will be amazed at how much sound affects the way we think, feel, and heal. I encourage you all to attend a sound bath. You never know what will surface after you move the energy. A few people to follow and check out include the band Shakti Tribe and sound bath artist Christian Reid (christianmichaelreid on Instagram). I find their healing frequencies to be life changing.

- **DNA/Human Design**: Study your DNA and personality to discover your place in this world. When you know who you are, how you are made, and what you represent, you know where to direct your energy and attention. Utilize Human

Design and the other personality tests in this book to access knowledge that could take you decades to figure out on your own. Put your print-outs in a three-ring binder, building your own human manual.

I recommend Dylan Varenhorst the spirit advisor, who has been studying and implementing Human Design for over a decade. His readings are unique to your DNA blueprint, and he offers one-on-one and group family readings you can record and listen to over and over to know your true path. You can connect to his website through my website, https://www.LuminaryHealingCenter.com.

- **Perfection**: There is no such thing as perfection. You will suffer needlessly if you attempt to achieve this in your lifetime. Accept that nothing is perfect, and you will free yourself to be imperfect.

- **Karma**: Karma is a good thing. It keeps teaching you until you get the lesson and learn from it. Clearing your karma is part of healing the soul. The goal is to redirect yourself when the issue comes up again. Conquer decisions with awareness and new directions, and you will eventually get it right. Clear up your karma, and you elevate to the next level.

- **Water**: Water is one of our most precious resources. Our bodies are made up of close to 70 percent water, so water is our cellular life force. Clean, living water will flush out toxins and bring in cellular healing, clarity, and alignment with true selves. I did the research and discovered the best natural-spring healing water filtration system. This is the system people with cancer and other illnesses turn to when they have been diagnosed. Why wait until then when you can have these healing waters now as a preventative measure?

Your entire family will benefit for the rest of their lives. And once you have it in your life, you will notice a difference in the way you think and feel and look. I am sharing all the healing techniques that are not talked about in mainstream healthcare because it is my soul purpose to teach people how to heal their bodies. Living water is health. You can access the water link at https://springaqua.info/wellnesswater or visit my website at https://www.LuminaryHealingCenter.com.

- **Air Purifier and Humidifier**: An air purifier can give your body clean, filtered air to breathe when you are sleeping, which we do for one-third of our lives. Adding a water humidifier puts moisture in the air, which is healthy for our skin and lungs. Doing whatever we can do to get our bodies functioning at their highest capacity and to heal while we rest will grant us longer, healthier lives.

- **Healthcare**: Holistic health is the present way to truly heal ourselves, our ancestors, and our future. We don't have to buy into a healthcare system that wants to pump us with drugs to make a profit and doesn't want us to realize we can create our very own good health. We can do this by working with holistic healthcare practitioners around the planet, thanks to the internet and Zoom. We need to dig in deep, access these rooted emotional layers, pull them up to the surface, clean them out, and process the data that has been stored in our central nervous system and cells in the body. No drug will take care of that. When you heal the body from the inside out, your chakras, meridians, and soul align, which in turn heals your organs, tissues, skin, and energy. You will radiate good health, and your aura will show it. People will notice and be drawn to you. Eventually, in this era of new earth, everyone will be able to see if someone has healed by the way they vibrate and radiate.

- **Intuition**: Your intuition develops as you get older and experience life. Energies and frequencies that you couldn't define suddenly become understandable, leading you to wisdom and knowledge from vibration alone. However, you have access to this information even at a young age. You can't quite determine what each frequency means just yet, but you can sense the frequencies.

Your gut, heart, body, feelings, emotions, and mind will give you clues. Pay attention to those details, and ask your body what it is trying to tell you. It will direct you if you are toxin-free and focused on listening and learning. You will receive messages through your third eye. You are not hearing strange voices; you are hearing divinely guided messages from your higher self. It sounds like a whisper. You may get a vision, hear a thought that seems odd: *Hello*—it's trying to get your attention.

We can get so sidetracked by all the commotion around us and what society has deemed normal. What I have learned is to always trust intuition. It is never wrong. Every time I write it off and ignore it, I learn this lesson all over again. Our bodies contain magnificent, invisible superpowers. We just have to learn how to tap in. When your body and soul is not on the right path, you will feel it. This misalignment will show up in sickness, life will not flow, and you will be met with resistance. Your intuition is your higher self leading the way.

- **Reset**: There are going to be times when you have to reset yourself: when you lose a pet, break off a relationship, change jobs, etc. Your body needs to go through a healing cycle to realign, and this kind of healing takes time. You don't want to jump into another relationship. There is a good chance you will recreate the same pattern you just got out of. You really need to dig in and clear the energy, evolve, and grow past it before you can move on in a healthy way.

  When doing a reset, go back to the basics of R to the eighth power, a.k.a. the eight Rs to soul healing. Nurture yourself with self-love, rest, sleep, nutritious foods, water, supplements, exercise, sunshine, activities you enjoy, and journaling to release. Your body needs to recover, move energy, and then recover and realign again. You will do this several times over as you move energy and heal needed gaps in the aura, soul, and body. This is how you heal the soul and body to gain momentum to excellent health, mindset, and wellness.

- **Therapists/Counselors/Coaches/Mentors/Healers**: We all need therapists, counselors, coaches, mentors, and healers throughout our journey of life. There is no way to know how to handle each situation that will be thrown at us. We must therefore empower ourselves with the best resources around the world, who can guide us to make good choices, come up with solutions, and offer suggestions.

- **Binders**: You are the master of your own destiny. You didn't come with an operating manual, but I have given you the tools to create your own. Use a three-ring binder to accumulate your personality data. Use a three-ring binder for your health data. Use a three-ring binder to compile data for your home, appliances, and big purchases. Hard copies are best to refer back to at any given time, should you not have access to a computer.

- **Electronic Files**: Electronic files are not private. Put any electronic files you wish to keep onto a backup resource, such as an external drive. Data is being stolen every day. Don't let your data be stolen and sold back to you or used against you.

- **Microchanneling**: We don't have to put overpriced toxins in the body or go to extremes to maintain our youthful glow. We can take the holistic approach and use a newer technique called microchanneling. Microchanneling is a needle-stamping technique vs. microneedling, in which a needle is dragged across the skin.

    I did the research and decided to become certified in microchanneling in order to show you a natural way for the body to repair itself and maintain a natural glow. If you see me online or meet me in person, I want you to know I have not had any plastic surgery (at least, not up until 2022, but I have learned never to say never), nor have I put toxic injections in my face for several years. Microchanneling enables the body to do what it does best: heal itself. Holistic health is our new earth.

If you would like to book an appointment to receive holistic microchanneling and a private healing consultation, connect through https://www.LuminaryHealingCenter.com.

- **PEMF/Pulsated Electromagnetic Field Therapy**: Technology will play a huge factor in the future of healing our bodies. PEMF therapy uses invisible light frequency, and since people can't see, hear, or feel it, it has been misunderstood and overlooked by many doctors.

    When using PEMF, I found the results to be profound. Some days I pooped twice, which is much harder to do when you get older, by the way. I know: TMI. But I gotta drive a point home here. Getting the poop out gets the toxins out. I am lighter and clearer. PEMF has helped with discomforts in my body, helped me get off medications, flushed out the blood in my body, and my mental functioning is so off the charts that I pretty much pounded out this book in a couple of months. Imagine what that would do for your test-taking capabilities. Heck, we should do a study on people who use PEMF and don't use PEMF and compare their results physically and mentally. But I bet someone has already done that.

    Professional athletes and sports teams use PEMF therapy. It's moving into colleges and, I hope, every household. Who wouldn't want to feel great every day? PEMF enhances vitality, well-being, sleep, stress reduction, relaxation, endurance, energy, nutrient and oxygen delivery, local blood flow, waste removal, muscle conditioning, athletic performance, muscle recovery, physical fitness, and strength. Can you imagine what this will do for the people in your family? Your grandparents?

Benefits also include helping the body's natural recovery process, correcting cellular dysfunction throughout the body, and stimulating and exercising cells to recharge them, thus giving humans more energy naturally. This one thing alone is a game changer. Hit up https://www.LuminaryHealingCenter.com to book a personal consultation.

- **Superpower Hour/Safe After-School Space**: Create a support group on campus after school with counselors. Gather together to journal in silence and release. The coming together of healing minds can have a very powerful impact. Dance to release energy and share positive energy; ground in the grass with no shoes, run in the sprinklers, eat superfoods (maybe get a health food sponsor). Students should get one-on-one time with a counselor, if only for fifteen minutes, to talk. Counselors can teach coping mechanisms, help students identify toxic behavior, and engender self-love and acceptance of other people's superpowers. We need healers of all kinds to make the world go round. If there is something you bring to the table, show it off.

- **Yoga**: Becoming a certified yoga instructor is pretty awesome. Teaching and modeling how to live a healthy life is a fantastic soul purpose.

- **Cycling**: Going cycling is a great way to burn off stress, move energy, and release. Start up a cycling club and see what happens. You could very well start a trend.

- **Meditation**: Teaching people to quiet their minds and go within is a needed superpower. As simple as it sounds, many people can't seem to take the time to meditate and master this trait. Sitting in silence with a group of people has a very profound healing effect. Your minds will intertwine, connecting energy, knowledge, and resources. When meditating on the grass under a tree, infinite knowledge can be accessed as a group. Meditation over medication any day.

- **Ascension**: Achieving energy activation of the rainbow light body, moving from the lower density of the third dimension to the fifth dimension and beyond. The path to ascension is unconditional love, acceptance, forgiveness, purity, natural perfection, holistic healing, angelic status and being.

## Great Tips

- Life is not about making money.
- Life is about positive energy exchange with one another.
- Compassion, forgiveness, and unconditional love unleash your superpowers.
- Health and happiness is the winning strategy.
- Health trumps wealth.
- How you make people feel is what they will remember.
- Radiate rainbows.
- The new earth is rebirth of the earth.
- Frequency heals DNA.
- Kindness is the master of keys to any castle, door, job, opportunity, and relationship.
- Kindness is an invisible superpower money can't buy.
- You create the most abundant energy exchange when you share it with the right people.
- Look for the good in people; give people compliments in order to have a positive energy exchange. Your vibration lifts and so does theirs.

- Social media is your reputation for life and your online résumé blueprint. If you don't have anything nice to say, don't say anything at all. Better yet, eliminate social media altogether, and your superpowers will soar. Keeping your life private and off social media will prevent it from being used against you. Social media hurts people on deep emotional and psychological levels. It opens the door to predators, scammers, and human traffickers and may very well be capturing fragments of your soul.
- The digital matrix is brain programming; beware.
- Sober activities are the best hangouts to raise your vibration. The library, board games, bowling, karaoke, bide rides, hiking, canoeing, and stand-up paddle boarding are great activities to do.

Always believe, in your soul, that you are indestructible.

# EPILOGUE

Be on the lookout for my next book. There is still *so* much more to share with you. Stay strong, keep clear, and you will see past the illusions. Every day, new schemes are being invented to try and grab your attention and fool you. Trust your gut. Trust your soul. Trust your higher self. It is always right.

Join us online at https://www.NoelleHipke.com for events to connect and learn from each other on how to develop your superpowers. Connect to me on LinkedIn, Instagram, FB, Twitter and YouTube. I'd love to hear from you and your thoughts about this book.

May you all be able to see the invisible now!

Welcome to ascension into another dimension: 3D to 5D is the new reality.

If you feel this book has brought you value or taught you something worthy of sharing, I would so be honored if you would take a few minutes to write me a book review on Amazon. You and your review will now become part of the worldwide movement to help humanity heal together. Welcome to the conscious community and the Great Awakening!

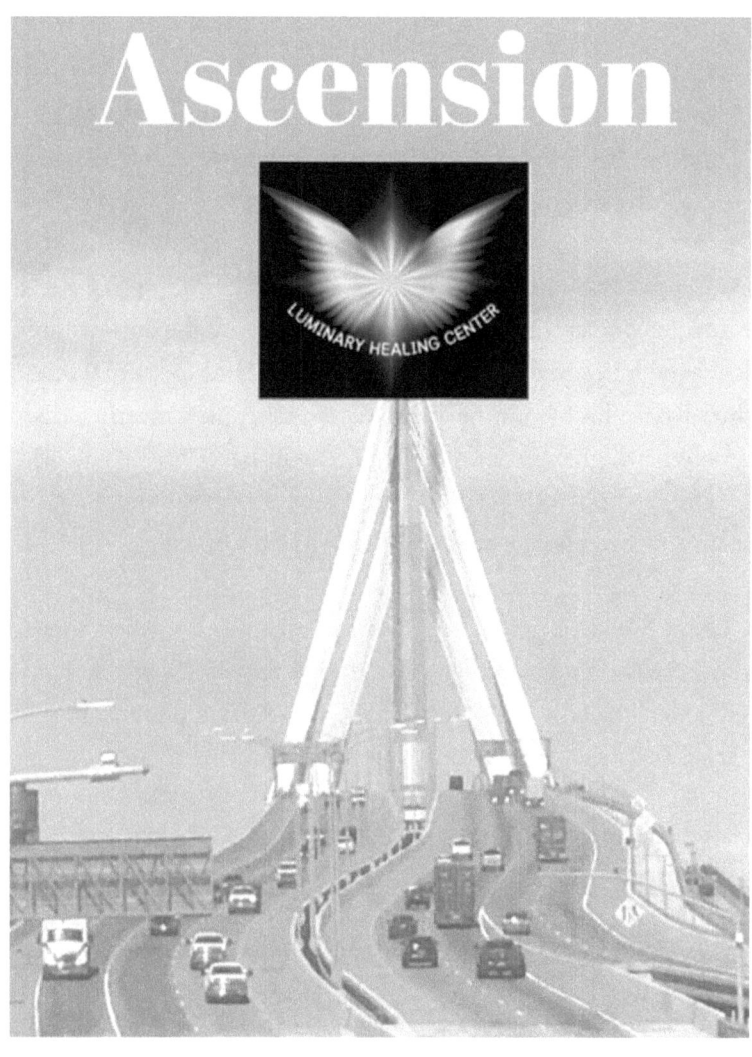

# ACKNOWLEDGMENTS

Gaia TV: Thank you for opening the door to the pathway of heaven and earth. Your programs inspire, educate, and give viewers something to contemplate.

Koehler Books and John Koehler: Gratitude to John Koehler and the Koehler Books team. Thank you for giving me the opportunity to upload my entire manuscript to your website and for contacting me within twenty-four-hours of the upload to schedule a meeting, discuss this book, and give me an offer. John, I will never forget you asking me, "Did anybody else help you write this book? You did good, girl. You are going to change so many lives with this book."

Larisa Stow: Larisa looked into my eyes when we first met and told me she was drawn to help me. Little did she know where that was going to lead or how much impact she would have on me and others for eternity. Larisa, you are one heck of a bright light.

TIG: The "Trust in God" man, who wishes to remain anonymous.

*I love you all.*

~Noelle Hipke

# REFERENCES

*The 4 DISC Personalities.* (2019, July 26). YouTube. https://www.youtube.com/watch?v=zuTSbiwFqOo

*2022 Science of Healing Summit.* (n.d.). Shift Network. Retrieved March 1, 2022, from https://scienceofhealingsummit.com/

*2022 Science of Healing Summit.* (2022, February 26). Shift Network. Retrieved February 26, 2022, from https://scienceofhealingsummit.com/

*About | 4BiddenKnowledge | Weston, FL United States.* (n.d.). 4BiddenKnowledge. Retrieved March 29, 2022, from https://www.4biddenknowledge.com/bio

About, A. (2022, May 10). *Universal Energy Flow Model - Population Dynamics.* Ecology Center. Retrieved March 31, 2022, from https://www.ecologycenter.us/population-dynamics-2/a-universal-energy-flow-model.html

*About Sound Baths.* (n.d.). Sound Baths & Yoga With Christian. Retrieved March 31, 2022, from http://soundbathsandyoga.com/about-sound-baths

*Accepting Miraculous Change.* (n.d.). Gaia Miraculous Change. Retrieved March 29, 2022, from https://www.gaia.com/video/accepting-miraculous-change?fullplayer=feature

*ADD vs ADHD.* (2016, December 2). WebMD. Retrieved March 8, 2022, from https://www.webmd.com/add-adhd/childhood-adhd/add-vs-adhd

Admin, A. (2021, October 26). *Symbolism - Examples and Definition of Symbolism.* Literary Devices. Retrieved March 10, 2022, from https://literarydevices.net/symbolism/

*Adult attention-deficit/hyperactivity disorder (ADHD) - Symptoms and causes.* (2019, June 22). Mayo Clinic. Retrieved March 8, 2022, from https://www.mayoclinic.org/diseases-conditions/adult-adhd/symptoms-causes/syc-20350878

*Alchemy & Imagination.* (n.d.). Gaia Alchemy Imagination. Retrieved April 15, 2022, from https://www.gaia.com/video/alchemy-imagination?fullplayer=feature

*Ancient Codes of History.* (n.d.). Gaia Ancient Codes of History. Retrieved March 29, 2022, from https://www.gaia.com/video/ancient-codes-of-history?fullplayer=feature

*Ancient meets Modern approach to achieving Optimal Health.* (2017, September 23). Alchemy Ayurveda. Retrieved March 29, 2022, from https://alchemyayurveda.com/my-approach/

*Ancient Technology of Ra.* (n.d.). Gaia. Retrieved April 21, 2022, from https://www.gaia.com/video/ancient-technology-ra?fullplayer=feature

Aor, A. (2016, October 6). *When did microwave ovens become very common in North American hom. . .* Fun Trivia. Retrieved March 23, 2022, from https://www.funtrivia.com/askft/Question3019.html

*Artificial Immortality.* (n.d.). Gaia. Retrieved May 19, 2022, from https://www.gaia.com/video/artificial-immortality?fullplayer=feature

*Awakening The Conscious Ego.* (n.d.). Gaia Awakening the Conscious Ego. Retrieved April 15, 2022, from https://www.gaia.com/video/awakening-the-conscious-ego?fullplayer=feature

Becker, D. G. (2000). *Protecting the Gift: Keeping Children and Teenagers Safe (and Parents Sane)* (Reprint). Dell.

Becker, D. G. (2021). *The Gift of Fear.* Back Bay Books.

*Becoming Supernatural with Joe Dispenza.* (n.d.). Gaia. Retrieved April 15, 2022, from https://www.gaia.com/video/becoming-supernatural-joe-dispenza?fullplayer=feature

*Biofield Tuning | A Sound Approach to Health & Well-being.* (n.d.). Biofieldtuning. Retrieved March 29, 2022, from https://www.biofieldtuning.com/

Bl, B. (2021, November 30). *Epigenetics.* Bruce H. Lipton, PhD. Retrieved March 29, 2022, from https://www.brucelipton.com/epigenetics/

*Blessing of the Energy Centers.* (n.d.). Gaia. Retrieved April 21, 2022, from https://www.gaia.com/video/blessing-energy-centers?fullplayer=feature

*Brain Crystals and Psychic Powers.* (n.d.). Gaia. Retrieved April 15, 2022, from https://www.gaia.com/video/brain-crystals-and-psychic-powers?fullplayer=feature

*Breaking Down ET Stereotypes.* (n.d.). Gaia. Retrieved April 15, 2022, from https://www.gaia.com/video/breaking-down-et-stereotypes?fullplayer=feature

*Breaking Emotional Patterns with Bill McKenna.* (n.d.). Gaia. Retrieved April 15, 2022, from https://www.gaia.com/video/breaking-emotional-patterns-bill-mckenna?fullplayer=feature

Brianna-Wiest, B. (2022, January 28). *20 Signs You're What's Known As A 'Lightworker.'* Thought Catalog. Retrieved March 29, 2022, from https://thoughtcatalog.com/brianna-wiest/2018/03/20-signs-youre-whats-known-as-a-lightworker/

Burnham, G., & Merrill, D. (2017). *The Gracia Burnham Collection: In the Presence of My Enemies / To Fly Again.* Tyndale House Publishers.

*Calling for Angelic Guidance with Joan Walker.* (n.d.). Gaia. Retrieved April 21, 2022, from https://www.gaia.com/video/calling-angelic-guidance-joan-walker?fullplayer=feature

Cameron, J. (2002). *The Artist's Way.* Van Haren Publishing.

*Channeling THEO: Soulful Relationships*. (n.d.). Gaia Channeling Theo. Retrieved April 15, 2022, from https://www.gaia.com/video/channeling-theo-soulful-relationships?fullplayer=feature

Cho, C. (2015). *The Little Book of Skin Care: Korean Beauty Secrets for Healthy, Glowing Skin* (First Edition). William Morrow.

Choquette, S. (1995). *The Psychic Pathway: A Workbook for Reawakening the Voice of Your

Soul*. Crown Publishing Group.

Christopher, J. (2014). *The Tripods Collection: The White Mountains; The City of Gold and Lead; The Pool of Fire; When the Tripods Came* (Boxed Set). Aladdin.

Coleman, W. L. (1996). *If I Could Raise My Kids Again* (First Edition). Bethany House Pub.

*Connecting With Universal Energy Flow – Brenda Rose*. (n.d.). Brenda Rose. Retrieved March 31, 2022, from https://www.brenda-rose.com/connecting-with-universal-energy-flow/Consciousreminder, C. (2017, October 23).

*There Are 12 Types Of Lightworkers That Transform The Human Spirit. Which One Are You?* Conscious Reminder. Retrieved March 29, 2022, from https://consciousreminder.com/2017/10/23/12-types-lightworkers-transform-human-spirit-one/

*Create Miracles*. (n.d.). Cognomovement. Retrieved March 29, 2022, from https://www.cognomovement.com/

Cronkleton, E. (2022, March 11). *What Are the Different Types of Massage?* Healthline. Retrieved March 31, 2022, from https://www.healthline.com/health/types-of-massage

Cymascope. (2022, February 3). *Home - Cymascope*. Cymascope - Cymatics and the Cymascope Device for Sound Research. Retrieved March 29, 2022, from https://cymascope.com/

Davenport, S. (2021, November 26). *5 of the best PEMF therapy devices for pain management.* Medical News Today. Retrieved March 23, 2022, from https://www.medicalnewstoday.com/articles/pemf-therapy-device

*David Elliott Healing Products.* (n.d.). David Elliott. Retrieved March 29, 2022, from https://www.davidelliott.com/

*David Wolfe: Detoxification — More Important than Nutrition.* (n.d.). Gaia David Wolfe Detoxification. Retrieved April 15, 2022, from https://www.gaia.com/video/david-wolfe-detoxification-more-important-nutrition?fullplayer=feature

*Density or Dimension?* (n.d.). Gaia Density or Dimension. Retrieved March 29, 2022, from https://www.gaia.com/video/density-or-dimension?fullplayer=feature

*Discover BEMER Technology: Vascular Therapy.* (n.d.). Bemer Group. Retrieved March 23, 2022, from https://united-states.bemergroup.com/en_us/human-line/home/

*Discover Music as Medicine.* (n.d.). The Shift Network. Retrieved February 28, 2022, from https://theshiftnetwork.com/Discover-Music-Medicine?utm_medium=affiliate&utm_source=infusionsoft&mc_cid=7609a7f844&mc_eid=c745a5df1f&affiliate=15464

*Discover Your Love Language - The 5 Love Languages®.* (n.d.). Northfield Publishing. Retrieved March 10, 2022, from https://www.5lovelanguages.com/

Dooley, M. (2016). *The Top Ten Things Dead People Want to Tell YOU* (Reprint). Hay House Inc.

*Dr. Masaru Emoto - Message from the Water.* (2019, July 14). [Video]. YouTube. https://www.youtube.com/watch?v=FTORSP3uNMA

*Dr. Wayne W. Dyer Podcast.* (2017, May 23). [Video]. iHeart. https://www.iheart.com/podcast/794-dr-wayne-w-dyer-podcast-29697930/

Duprey, D. (2021, March 5). *What Are Totem Animals?* YourTango. Retrieved March 10, 2022, from https://www.yourtango.com/2020334330/what-are-totem-animals-list-spirituality

*Earn Your Happy Podcast.* (2016, February 25). [Video]. Lori Harder. https://loriharder.com/podcast/

*Ecosystem In a Box - Spring Aqua.* (n.d.). Wellness Water. Retrieved November 20, 2021, from https://springaqua.com/wellnesswater

Ehrlich, R. (2021, September 6). *Dr. Bruce Lipton - A New Hope: Epigenetics and the Subconscious Mind.* Dr Ron Ehrlich. Retrieved March 31, 2022, from https://drronehrlich.com/dr-bruce-lipton-a-new-hope-epigenetics-and-the-subconscious-mind-2/

*Electromagnetic Fields and Cancer.* (2019, January 3). National Cancer Institute. Retrieved April 1, 2022, from https://www.cancer.gov/about-cancer/causes-prevention/risk/radiation/electromagnetic-fields-fact-sheet

*Emotional Abuse: Definitions, Signs, Symptoms, Examples | HealthyPlace.* (2021, December 17). Healthy Place. Retrieved March 8, 2022, from https://www.healthyplace.com/abuse/emotional-psychological-abuse/emotional-abuse-definitions-signs-symptoms-examples

*Energy Secrets of the Great Pyramid.* (n.d.). Gaia. Retrieved April 21, 2022, from https://www.gaia.com/video/energy-secrets-of-the-great-pyramid?fullplayer=feature

*Enlightenment.* (n.d.). Gaia. Retrieved April 15, 2022, from https://www.gaia.com/video/enlightenment?fullplayer=feature

*Entering the Dimension of Magic.* (n.d.). Gaia Dimension of Magic. Retrieved March 29, 2022, from https://www.gaia.com/video/entering-the-dimension-of-magic?fullplayer=feature

Environmental Working Group. 2005. Body Burden: The Pollution in Newborns. Washington, DC. Available online at https://www.ewg.org/ research/body-burden-pollution-newborns

*Eridu: City of Gods*. (n.d.). Gaia Eridu City of Gods. Retrieved April 15, 2022, from https://www.gaia.com/video/eridu-city-of-gods?fullplayer=feature

*Everything is Energy*. (n.d.). Gaia Everything Energy. Retrieved March 29, 2022, from https://www.gaia.com/video/everything-energy?fullplayer=feature

*Exploring Extrasensory Consciousness*. (n.d.). Gaia Exploring Extrasensory. Retrieved April 15, 2022, from https://www.gaia.com/video/exploring-extrasensory-consciousness?fullplayer=feature

*Extraterrestrial Races*. (n.d.). Gaia Extraterrestrial Races. Retrieved March 29, 2022, from https://www.gaia.com/video/extraterrestrial-races?fullplayer=feature

*Fat, Sick and Nearly Dead*. (2019, December 13). [Video]. YouTube. https://www.youtube.com/watch?v=q1z5WjjVL5c

*Free personality test, type descriptions, relationship and career advice | 16Personalities*. (n.d.). 16 Personalities. Retrieved March 10, 2022, from https://www.16personalities.com/

Friedlander, J., & Hemsher, G. (2012). *Basic Psychic Development: A User's Guide to Auras, Chakras & Clairvoyance* (Reprint). Weiser Books.

*Gaia - Conscious Media, Streaming Yoga Videos & More*. (n.d.). Gaia. Retrieved March 29, 2022, from https://www.gaia.com/

Gene Keys Publishing. (2022, September 17). *Home*. Gene Keys. Retrieved September 27, 2022, from https://genekeys.com/

Gregor, G. (n.d.). *Take the Free Enneagram Personality Test*. Personality Path. Retrieved March 10, 2022, from https://personalitypath.com/free-enneagram-personality-test/

*Hacking of the 3D Matrix*. (n.d.). Gaia Hacking of the 3D Matrix. Retrieved March 29, 2022, from https://www.gaia.com/video/hacking-of-the-3d-matrix?fullplayer=feature

*Hacking the Financial Matrix*. (n.d.). Gaia Hacking the Financial Matrix. Retrieved April 15, 2022, from https://www.gaia.com/video/hacking-the-financial-matrix?fullplayer=feature

*happiness podcast with dr. robert puff - Zoeken*. (2011, May 9). [Video]. YouTube. https://www.bing.com/search?q=happiness+podcast+with+dr.+robert+puff&cvid=9110da123acd4814ab88c3d22873b21f&aqs=edge.69i57.8639j0j4&FORM=ANAB01&PC=EDGEDB

*Heal*. (n.d.). Gaia. Retrieved January 5, 2022, from https://www.gaia.com/video/heal?fullplayer=feature

Healing, D. (2021, June 22). *The Emotion Code | Energy Healing Method*. Discover Healing. Retrieved March 29, 2022, from https://discoverhealing.com/the-emotion-code/

Healing, D. (2022, January 14). *The Body Code | Energy Healing Tips*. Discover Healing. Retrieved March 29, 2022, from https://discoverhealing.com/the-body-code/

*Healing Dreams with Robert Moss*. (n.d.). Gaia. Retrieved April 15, 2022, from https://www.gaia.com/video/healing-dreams-robert-moss?fullplayer=feature

*Healing with Lucid Dreaming*. (n.d.). Gaia. Retrieved April 15, 2022, from https://www.gaia.com/video/healing-with-lucid-dreaming?fullplayer=feature

Hipskind, J. (1998, April 8). *Palmistry: The Whole View* (2nd ed.). Llewellyn Publications.

holisticMain, h. (2022, May 4). *Muscle Testing And Therapy*. My Holistic Therapy. Retrieved March 29, 2022, from https://myholistictherapy.org/muscle-testing-and-therapy/

*Home :: ColorCode Personality Science*. (n.d.). Color Code. Retrieved March 10, 2022, from https://www.colorcode.com//

*Human Design: Discover Your Purpose with Richard Beaumont*. (n.d.). Gaia. Retrieved April 21, 2022, from https://www.gaia.

com/video/human-design-discover-your-purpose-richard-beaumont?fullplayer=feature

Hurst, K. (2017, May 23). *Numerology Report: The Secret Meaning Of Numbers 0 To 9*. The Law of Attraction. Retrieved March 10, 2022, from https://www.thelawofattraction.com/meanings-numbers-0-9/

*hypnosis | Definition, History, Techniques, & Facts*. (n.d.). Encyclopedia Britannica. Retrieved March 31, 2022, from https://www.britannica.com/science/hypnosis

*Hypnosis History*. (n.d.). John Mongiovi. Retrieved March 31, 2022, from https://johnmongiovi.com/history-hypnosis

*impact theory podcast - Zoeken*. (2017, January 4). [Video]. YouTube. https://www.bing.com/search?q=impact+theory+podcast&cvid=92538a4b1cd040b4871cb02764169f9a&aqs=edge.0.0j69i57j0l3j69i64.3695j0j4&FORM=ANAB01&PC=EDGEDB

*Initial Matrix vs. False Matrix*. (n.d.). Gaia Matrix Vs. False Matrix. Retrieved March 29, 2022, from https://www.gaia.com/video/initial-matrix-vs-false-matrix?fullplayer=feature

*An Inspired Life with Regina Meredith*. (n.d.). Gaia. Retrieved April 15, 2022, from https://www.gaia.com/video/inspired-life-regina-meredith?fullplayer=feature

*The Intelligent Heart*. (n.d.). Gaia. Retrieved April 21, 2022, from https://www.gaia.com/video/the-intelligent-heart?fullplayer=feature

*Intergalactic Organization Revealed*. (n.d.). Gaia. Retrieved April 15, 2022, from https://www.gaia.com/video/intergalactic-organization-revealed?fullplayer=feature

*Interstellar Highways: Portals & Toroids*. (n.d.). Gaia Intersteller Portals. Retrieved March 29, 2022, from https://www.gaia.com/video/interstellar-highways-portals-toroids?fullplayer=feature

*Iron deficiency anemia - Symptoms and causes.* (2022, January 4). Mayo Clinic. Retrieved February 22, 2022, from https://www.mayoclinic.org/diseases-conditions/iron-deficiency-anemia/symptoms-causes/syc-20355034

Jordan, T., MD (2016, October 18). *Podcast* [Video]. Dr. Tim Jordan. https://drtimjordan.com/category/podcast/

*Jovian Archive.* (n.d.). JovianArchive.com. Retrieved March 10, 2022, from https://www.jovianarchive.com/Human_Design/What_is_it

Joyner, S. (2021, February 9). *STEAM Education: Preparing All Students for the Future.* ViewSonic Library. Retrieved February 24, 2022, from https://www.viewsonic.com/library/education/steam-education-preparing-all-students-for-the-future/

Karrel, D. (2019). *Mastering the Basics.* McGraw-Hill Education.

Kelly, A. (2022, April 15). *What Master Numbers 11, 22 & 33 Mean In Numerology.* YourTango. Retrieved March 10, 2022, from https://www.yourtango.com/2018311236/astrology-what-does-master-numbers-mean-personality-traits-numerology-zodiac-signs

Kubala, M. J. S. (2018, November 14). *Zinc: Everything You Need to Know.* Healthline. Retrieved February 22, 22 C.E., from https://www.healthline.com/nutrition/zinc

Kubala, M. J. S. (2019, August 20). *7 Science-Based Health Benefits of Selenium.* Healthline. Retrieved February 22, 2022 from https://www.healthline.com/nutrition/selenium-benefits

Leech, M. J. S. (2018, October 5). *10 Health Benefits of Spirulina.* Healthline. Retrieved February 22, 2022, from https://www.healthline.com/nutrition/10-proven-benefits-of-spirulina#TOC_TITLE_HDR_4

*Leftyfretz: The Left Handed Guitar Player's Resource.* Retrieved March 24, 2023. https://leftyfretz.com/how-many-people-are-left-handed/

https://leftyfretz.com/25-facts-about-left-handed-people/

*Life Beyond Death*. (n.d.). Gaia Life Beyond Death. Retrieved March 29, 2022, from https://www.gaia.com/video/life-beyond-death?fullplayer=feature

Lindberg, S. (2020, August 24). *What Are the 7 Chakras and How Can You Unblock Them?* Healthline. Retrieved March 29, 2022, from https://www.healthline.com/health/what-are-chakras#the-7-main-chakras

*Linking Symbology Through Time*. (n.d.). Gaia. Retrieved April 15, 2022, from https://www.gaia.com/video/linking-symbology-through-time?fullplayer=feature

*Listening to Your Guides with Sonia Choquette*. (n.d.). Gaia. Retrieved April 21, 2022, from https://www.gaia.com/video/listening-your-guides-sonia-choquette?fullplayer=feature

Lwa0J, L. (2021, April 17). *History Of Essential Oils*. Essential Oils Academy. Retrieved March 31, 2022, from https://essentialoilsacademy.com/history/

*Matrix Manipulations from the Moon*. (n.d.). Gaia Matrix Manipulations From the Moon. Retrieved March 29, 2022, from https://www.gaia.com/video/matrix-manipulations-from-the-moon?fullplayer=feature

*Measurement of the Human Biofield and Other Energetic Instruments*. (n.d.). Foundation for Alternative and Integrative Medicine. Retrieved February 28, 2022, from https://www.faim.org/measurement-of-the-human-biofield-and-other-energetic-instruments

Microphones, D. (2021, March 3). *Facts about speech intelligibility: human voice frequency range*. DPA. Retrieved March 31, 2022, from https://www.dpamicrophones.com/mic-university/facts-about-speech-intelligibility

Morelli, K. (2022, January 31). *Home*. Bruce H. Lipton, PhD. Retrieved March 29, 2022, from https://www.brucelipton.com/

*The Mystical Experience: Wisdom From the Plant Teachers | 2022 Science of Healing Summit.* (n.d.). The Shift Network. Retrieved February 28, 2022, from https://scienceofhealingsummit.com/program/46729

Nedasaleh, N. (2018, January 15). *12 Benefits of Detoxing the Body.* Evoke Acupuncture. Retrieved February 22, 2022, from https://evokeacupuncture.com/12-benefits-of-detoxing-the-body/

Network, T. (n.d.-a). *A Conversation With Deepak Chopra, MD & Anoop Kumar, MD on Quantum Healing | 2022 Science of Healing Summit.* The Shift Network. Retrieved March 2, 2022, from https://scienceofhealingsummit.com/program/46614

Network, T. (n.d.-b). *Coherence: How to Get in Sync With Your Higher Self, Others, and the Earth | 2022 Science of Healing Summit.* The Shift Network. Retrieved March 3, 2022, from https://scienceofhealingsummit.com/program/46328

Network, T. (n.d.-c). *Energy, the Biofield, and Personal Healing | 2022 Science of Healing Summit.* The Shift Network. https://scienceofhealingsummit.com/program/46977

Network, T. (n.d.-d). *Essentials of Medical Intuition: A Visionary Path to Wellness | 2022 Science of Healing Summit.* The Shift Network. Retrieved March 6, 2022, from https://scienceofhealingsummit.com/program/47258

Network, T. (n.d.-e). *Growing a New Body: Healing by Detoxification | 2022 Science of Healing Summit.* The Shift Network. Retrieved March 1, 2022, from https://scienceofhealingsummit.com/program/47027

Network, T. (n.d.-f). *Healing as Intended | 2022 Science of Healing Summit.* The Shift Network. Retrieved March 3, 2022, from https://scienceofhealingsummit.com/program/47022

Network, T. (n.d.-g). *Healing Within: Energy Psychology Treatment for Trauma | 2022 Science of Healing Summit.* The Shift Network.

Retrieved March 5, 2022, from https://scienceofhealingsummit.com/program/47018

Network, T. (n.d.-h). *Lower Your Risk of COVID & Help Yourself Overcome Long-Haul COVID | 2022 Science of Healing Summit.* The Shift Network. Retrieved March 5, 2022, from https://scienceofhealingsummit.com/program/46654

Network, T. (n.d.-i). *Psychedelics and Mental Health | 2022 Science of Healing Summit.* The Shift Network. Retrieved March 2, 2022, from https://scienceofhealingsummit.com/program/46734

Network, T. (n.d.-j). *Shift Talk: The Future of Mental Wellness — It's Not What You Think | 2022 Science of Healing Summit.* The Shift Network. Retrieved March 3, 2022, from https://scienceofhealingsummit.com/program/46657

Network, T. (n.d.-k). *The Awakening Potential in Trauma: A Calling to Self-Actualize | 2022 Science of Healing Summit.* The Shift Network. Retrieved March 5, 2022, from https://scienceofhealingsummit.com/program/46557

Network, T. (n.d.-l). *The Wisdom Behind the Wisdom Codes | 2022 Science of Healing Summit.* The Shift Network. Retrieved March 1, 2022, from https://scienceofhealingsummit.com/program/46853

Network, T. (n.d.-m). *What Does Personal Self-Integration Have to Do With Healing | 2022 Science of Healing Summit.* The Shift Network. Retrieved March 4, 2022, from https://scienceofhealingsummit.com/program/46660

Numerology.com. (n.d.). *Numerology.com – Free Daily Numerology, Numerology readings, Numerology compatibility, and more.* Retrieved March 10, 2022, from https://www.numerology.com/

Numerology.com Staff. (2021, October 18). *Number 4 Meaning.* Numerology.com. Retrieved March 10, 2022, from https://www.numerology.com/articles/about-numerology/single-digit-number-4-meaning/

*The Official Website of Billy Carson | 4BiddenKnowledge | Weston, FL USA*. (n.d.). 4BiddenKnowledge. Retrieved March 29, 2022, from https://www.4biddenknowledge.com/

Olsen, R. N. D. (2018, September 17). *Selenium Deficiency*. Healthline. Retrieved February 22, 2022, from https://www.healthline.com/health/selenium-deficiency

*OMNIUM UNIVERSE*. (n.d.). Omnium Universe. Retrieved March 29, 2022, from https://www.omniumuniverse.com/

Orloff, J. (2018). *The Empath's Survival Guide: Life Strategies for Sensitive People* (Reprint). Sounds True.

*Otherworldly Connections to Megaliths with Freddy Silva*. (n.d.). Gaia. Retrieved April 21, 2022, from https://www.gaia.com/video/otherworldly-connections-megaliths-freddy-silva?fullplayer=feature

*Passive-aggressive behavior: What are the red flags?* (2021, December 15). Mayo Clinic. Retrieved March 8, 2022, from https://www.mayoclinic.org/healthy-lifestyle/adult-health/expert-answers/passive-aggressive-behavior/faq-20057901

*A Path to 5D Ascension*. (n.d.). Gaia Ascension. Retrieved March 29, 2022, from https://www.gaia.com/video/a-path-to-5d-ascension?fullplayer=feature

Ph.D., H. (2010). *Loyalty To Your Soul: The Heart of Spiritual Psychology by Hulnick Ph.D., H. Ronald, Hulnick Ph.D., Mary R. [Hay House, 2011] (Paperback) [Paperback]*. Hay House,2011.

*Physiognomy or Face reading body language and how to read different types of faces*. (n.d.). Retrieved September 27, 2022, from https://askastrologer.com/Physiognomy.html

*Pineal Gland & the Quantum Field*. (n.d.). Gaia. Retrieved April 15, 2022, from https://www.gaia.com/video/pineal-gland-quantum-field?fullplayer=feature

*Podcast*. (2017, January 10). [Video]. The Cathy Heller Show. https://www.dontkeepyourdayjob.com/podcast/

*Podcast | LOVE Life | How to Get the Guy.* (2015, December 2). [Video]. Get the Guy. https://www.howtogettheguy.com/podcast/

*Podcast Archive.* (2017, January 25). [Video]. Melissa Ambrosini. https://melissaambrosini.com/podcast/

MD, PhD H (2002) *Power vs.Force: The Hidden Determinants of Human Behavior* by David R. Hawkins MD, PhD.[Hay House, 2002] (Paperback) Hay House, 2002

*Portals, Stargates, & Time Travel.* (n.d.). Gaia. Retrieved April 21, 2022, from https://www.gaia.com/video/portals-stargates-time-travel?fullplayer=feature

Prout, S. (2020, January 27). *7 Signs You're A True Lightworker*. Sarah Prout. Retrieved March 29, 2022, from https://sarahprout.com/signs-you-are-a-lightworker/

Psychology Tools. (2022, May 17). *Fight Or Flight Response*. Retrieved March 8, 2022, from https://www.psychologytools.com/resource/fight-or-flight-response/

*Purium - The Transformation Company Corporate Site.* (n.d.). Purium. Retrieved February 22, 2022, from https://ishoppurium.com/

*Quantum Communication: Part 2.* (n.d.). Gaia. Retrieved April 21, 2022, from https://www.gaia.com/video/quantum-communication-part-2?fullplayer=feature

*Quantum Uncertainty.* (n.d.). Gaia Quantum Uncertainty. Retrieved March 29, 2022, from https://www.gaia.com/video/quantum-uncertainty?fullplayer=feature

*Quick Coherence.* (n.d.). Gaia. Retrieved April 15, 2022, from https://www.gaia.com/video/quick-coherence?fullplayer=feature

Ramaswamy, S., Ramaswamy, S., & Ramaswamy, S. (2021, June 26). *Alchemy Ayurveda - Mind. Body. Spirit. Transformation.*

Alchemy Ayurveda. Retrieved March 29, 2022, from https://alchemyayurveda.com/

Redfield, J., & Adrienne, C. (1995). *The Celestine Prophecy: An Experiential Guide* (Illustrated). Warner Books.

*Redirecting Timelines.* (n.d.). Gaia Redirecting Timelines. Retrieved March 29, 2022, from https://www.gaia.com/video/redirecting-timelines?fullplayer=feature

*Reptilian Installations on Earth.* (n.d.). Gaia. Retrieved April 18, 2022, from https://www.gaia.com/video/reptilian-installations-on-earth?fullplayer=feature

Riley, S., Riley, S., Riley, S., Riley, S., Harris, T., Riley, S., Maslyk, J., Branstetter, D., Sandstrom, B., Riley, S., Grundler, M. A. L., Petris, D., Longo, S., Hodson, L., & Simmons, M. (n.d.). *STEAM Archives.* The Institute for Arts Integration and STEAM. Retrieved February 24, 2022, from https://artsintegration.com/topics/approaches/steam/

Roberts, G. L. (2017, May 23). *What are the benefits of emotional intelligence? - Developing Your Emotional Intelligence.* LinkedIn. Retrieved April 11, 2020, from https://www.linkedin.com/learning/developing-your-emotional-intelligence/what-are-the-benefits-of-emotional-intelligence?

Rosen, B. R. (2010, June 11). *Developing Your 5 Clair Senses - Rebecca Rosen.* Oprah.com. Retrieved April 1, 2022, from https://www.oprah.com/spirit/developing-your-5-clair-senses-rebecca-rosen/all

Ruiz, D. M. (1997). *The Four Agreements: A Practical Guide to Personal Freedom (A Toltec Wisdom Book).* Amber-Allen Publishing, Incorporated.

*Sacred Geometry: Spiritual Science* (n.d.). Gaia. Retrieved March 23, 2023, fromhttps://www.gaia.com/series/sacred-geometry-spiritual-science

Sahara Rose. (2022, May 5). *The Highest Self Podcast* [with video]. Sahara Rose. https://iamsahararose.com/podcast/

*The Science of the Heart.* (n.d.). Gaia. Retrieved April 15, 2022, from https://www.gaia.com/video/science-heart?fullplayer=feature

*Self-Healing Through Vedic Astrology.* (n.d.). Gaia Self-Healing Through Vedic Astrology. Retrieved April 15, 2022, from https://www.gaia.com/video/self-healing-through-vedic-astrology?fullplayer=feature

*Sensitive: The Untold Story.* (n.d.). Gaia. Retrieved April 21, 2022, from https://www.gaia.com/video/sensitive-untold-story?fullplayer=feature

*Seven Symbols of Atlantis.* (n.d.). Gaia. Retrieved April 15, 2022, from https://www.gaia.com/video/seven-symbols-atlantis?fullplayer=feature

Sherrell, Z. M. (2022a, January 31). *What to know about biofield therapy.* Medical News Today. Retrieved March 8, 2022, from https://www.medicalnewstoday.com/articles/biofield-therapy

Sherrell, Z. M. (2022b, January 31). *What to know about biofield therapy.* Medical News Today. Retrieved April 1, 2022, from https://www.medicalnewstoday.com/articles/biofield-therapy

*Shifting into Higher States of Being.* (n.d.). Gaia Shifting Higher State of Being. Retrieved April 15, 2022, from https://www.gaia.com/video/shifting-higher-states-being?fullplayer=feature

*Shows.* (2016, February 10). [Video]. Earth Speak. https://www.earthspeak.love/shows

*A Simple Method for Manifestation.* (n.d.). Gaia. Retrieved April 21, 2022, from https://www.gaia.com/video/a-simple-method-for-manifestation?fullplayer=feature

*A Simple Method for Profound Healing with Bill McKenna.* (n.d.). Gaia. Retrieved April 15, 2022, from https://www.gaia.com/video/simple-method-profound-healing-bill-mckenna?fullplayer=feature

Sloan, E. (2021, July 13). *Here's What Each Planet Actually Means in Astrology—So You Can Understand Your Chart in More Depth.* Well+Good. Retrieved March 10, 2022, from https://www.wellandgood.com/meanings-of-planets-in-astrology/

*SoulTalk with Kute Blackson.* (2018, January 24). [Video]. YouTube. http://podcast.kuteblackson.com/

*Sound & Megaliths.* (n.d.). Gaia Sound Megaliths. Retrieved March 29, 2022, from https://www.gaia.com/video/sound-megaliths?fullplayer=feature

*Sound Throughout Time.* (n.d.). Gaia. Retrieved March 29, 2022, from https://www.gaia.com/video/sound-throughout-time?fullplayer=feature

*Stay Inspired: Harmonizing Your Heart and Brain with Gregg Braden.* (n.d.). Gaia. Retrieved April 15, 2022, from https://www.gaia.com/video/stay-inspired-harmonizing-your-heart-and-brain-gregg-braden?fullplayer=feature

Stern, R. (n.d.). *Gaslighting in relationships: How to spot it and shut it down.* Vox. Retrieved May 1, 2022, from https://www.vox.com/first-person/2018/12/19/18140830/gaslighting-relationships-politics-explained

Stow, L. (2019, November 6). *Why Slay Dragons When You Can Ride Them?* Larisa Stow and Shakti Tribe. Retrieved March 29, 2022, from https://larisastow.com/

*The Super Soul Podcast - Listen & Subscribe | OWN.* (2017, January 27). [Video]. Oprah.com. https://www.oprah.com/app/super-soul-podcast.html

*Taking Your Place in the Universe with Steven Ross.* (n.d.). Gaia Taking Your Place. Retrieved April 15, 2022, from https://www.gaia.com/video/taking-your-place-universe-steven-ross?fullplayer=feature

*Time Wars & Progenitor ET Influences.* (n.d.). Gaia. Retrieved April 19, 2022, from https://www.gaia.com/video/time-wars-progenitor-et-influences?fullplayer=feature

*Transcending Genetic Tampering.* (n.d.). Gaia Genetic Tampering. Retrieved March 29, 2022, from https://www.gaia.com/video/transcending-genetic-tampering?fullplayer=feature

*Type Descriptions.* (n.d.). The Enneagram Institute. Retrieved March 10, 2022, from https://www.enneaграminstitute.com/type-descriptions

*Unconscious - Definition, Meaning & Synonyms.* (n.d.). Vocabulary.com. Retrieved March 8, 2022, from https://www.vocabulary.com/dictionary/unconscious

*Understanding & Using Bioenergetic Medicine.* (n.d.). Gaia Bioenergetic Medicine. Retrieved March 29, 2022, from https://www.gaia.com/video/understanding-using-bioenergetic-medicine?fullplayer=feature

*Using the Emotion Code to Ease Suffering with Bradley Nelson.* (n.d.). Gaia Using Emotion Code Bradley Nelson. Retrieved April 15, 2022, from https://www.gaia.com/video/using-emotion-code-ease-suffering-bradley-nelson?fullplayer=feature

*Victims of Sexual Violence: Statistics | RAINN.* (n.d.). Rainn. Retrieved March 8, 2022, from https://www.rainn.org/statistics/victims-sexual-violence

Vrabec, S. (n.d.). *Water is Magic.* Pinterest. Retrieved February 22, 2022, from https://www.pinterest.com/yanetis/water-is-magic/

Walle, M. G. S. van de. (2019, March 11). *Full Body Detox: 9 Ways to Rejuvenate Your Body.* Healthline. Retrieved February 22, 2022, from https://www.healthline.com/nutrition/how-to-detox-your-body

Ware, M. R. (2017, October 23). *Health benefits and risks of copper.* Medical News Today. Retrieved February 22, 22 C.E., from https://www.medicalnewstoday.com/articles/288165#effects_of_deficiency

Warren, R. (2002). *The Purpose Driven Life: What on Earth Am I Here For? 40 Days of Purpose Campaign Edition* (1st ed.). Zondervan Press.

Woodward Thomas, K. (2004). *Calling In The One: 7 Weeks to Attract the Love of Your Life.* Penguin Random House

*The Way of Miracles.* (n.d.). Gaia the Way of Miracles. Retrieved April 15, 2022, from https://www.gaia.com/video/the-way-of-miracles?fullplayer=feature

*What Are the Basic Principles of Feng Shui?* (2021, January 26). The Spruce. Retrieved March 31, 2022, from https://www.thespruce.com/what-is-feng-shui-1275060

*What Is Reiki?* (2017, June 4). WebMD. Retrieved March 31, 2022, from https://www.webmd.com/pain-management/reiki-overview

*What is the difference between the pituitary gland and the pineal gland? | Socratic.* (n.d.). Socratic.org. Retrieved February 22, 2022, from https://socratic.org/questions/what-is-the-difference-between-the-pituitary-gland-and-the-pineal-gland

*What is the DiSC assessment?* (n.d.). Discprofile.com. Retrieved March 10, 2022, from https://www.discprofile.com/what-is-disc

White, A. (2020, June 22). *11 Benefits of Burning Sage, How to Get Started, and More.* Healthline. Retrieved March 31, 2022, from https://www.healthline.com/health/benefits-of-burning-sage

*Who Are the Taygetans?* (n.d.). Gaia. Retrieved April 11, 2022, from https://www.gaia.com/video/who-are-the-taygetans?fullplayer=feature

*Who Owns Ancestry.com? Everything You Need to Know.* (2022, February 7). Smarter Hobby. Retrieved March 10, 2022, from https://www.smarterhobby.com/genealogy/who-owns-ancestry/

Wikipedia contributors. (2022a, April 16). *The Tripods*. Wikipedia. Retrieved May 27, 2022, from https://en.wikipedia.org/wiki/The_Tripods

Wikipedia contributors. (2022b, May 12). *Masaru Emoto*. Wikipedia. Retrieved February 22, 2022, from https://en.wikipedia.org/wiki/Masaru_Emoto

*Will vs. Trust: What's the Difference?* (2022, May 17). Investopedia. Retrieved March 8, 2022, from https://www.investopedia.com/articles/personal-finance/051315/will-vs-trust-difference-between-two.asp

www.ingramcontent.com/pod-product-compliance
Lightning Source LLC
Chambersburg PA
CBHW060349080526
44583CB00012B/236